Understanding
Childhood
Eczema

Understanding Illness and Health

Many health problems and worries are strongly influenced by our thoughts and feelings. These exciting new books, written by experts in the psychology of health, are essential reading for sufferers, their families and friends.

Each book presents objective, easily understood information and advice about what the problem is, the treatments available and, most importantly, how your state of mind can help or hinder the way you cope. You will discover how to have a positive, hopeful outlook, which will help you choose the most effective treatment for you and your particular lifestyle, with confidence.

The series is edited by JANE OGDEN, Reader in Health Psychology, Guy's, King's and St Thomas' School of Medicine, King's College London, UK

Titles in the series

KAREN BALLARD Understanding Menopause

SIMON DARNLEY & BARBARA MILLAR Understanding Irritable Bowel Syndrome

LINDA PAPADOPOULOS & CARL WALKER Understanding Skin Problems

PENNY TITMAN Understanding Childhood Eczema

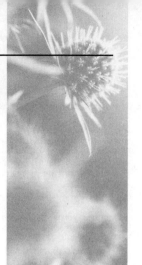

Understanding Childhood Eczema

PENNY TITMAN

Consultant Clinical Psychologist

WILEY

Copyright © 2003   John Wiley & Sons Ltd, The Atrium, Southern Gate, Chichester,
West Sussex PO19 8SQ, England

Telephone (+44) 1243 779777

Email (for orders and customer service enquiries): cs-books@wiley.co.uk
Visit our Home Page on www.wileyeurope.com or www.wiley.com

This publication is designed to provide accurate and authoritative information in regard to the subject
matter covered. It is sold on the understanding that the Publisher is not engaged in rendering
professional services. If professional advice or other expert assistance is required, the services of a
competent professional should be sought.

Other Wiley Editorial Offices

John Wiley & Sons Inc., 111 River Street, Hoboken, NJ 07030, USA

Jossey-Bass, 989 Market Street, San Francisco, CA 94103-1741, USA

Wiley-VCH Verlag GmbH, Boschstr. 12, D-69469 Weinheim, Germany

John Wiley & Sons Australia Ltd, 33 Park Road, Milton, Queensland 4064, Australia

John Wiley & Sons (Asia) Pte Ltd, 2 Clementi Loop #02-01, Jin Xing Distripark, Singapore 129809

John Wiley & Sons Canada Ltd, 22 Worcester Road, Etobicoke, Ontario, Canada M9W 1L1

Wiley also publishes its books in a variety of electronic formats. Some content that appears
in print may not be available in electronic books.

Library of Congress Cataloging-in-Publication Data

Titman, Penny.
  Understanding childhood eczema / Penny Titman.
      p. ; cm. – (Understanding illness and health)
Includes bibliographical references and index.
  ISBN 0-470-84759-X (paper : alk. paper)
 1. Eczema in children – Popular works.
  [DNLM: 1. Eczema – therapy – Popular Works. 2.
Eczema – psychology – Popular Works.   WR 190 T619u 2003]   I. Title. II.
Understanding illness & health.
  RJ516.E35T55 2003
  618.92′521 – dc21

                                                                2003001376

British Library Cataloguing in Publication Data

A catalogue record for this book is available from the British Library

ISBN 0-470-84759-X

Illustrations by Jason Broadbent

Typeset in 9.5/13pt Photina by Laserwords Private Limited, Chennai, India
Printed and bound in Great Britain by TJ International Ltd, Padstow, Cornwall
This book is printed on acid-free paper responsibly manufactured from sustainable forestry
in which at least two trees are planted for each one used for paper production.

Contents

About the author

DR PENNY TITMAN trained as a clinical psychologist at University College London and has since specialised in working with children and their families. She has extensive experience of working with children with physical health problems, including skin conditions, as well as in child mental health services. Dr Titman carried out a special study of the impact of eczema and other skin conditions on the wellbeing of children and families and this work formed the basis of her PhD. She currently works as a consultant clinical psychologist in a community team for children and families in an NHS Trust.

Acknowledgements

I am very grateful to Dr Jane Ogden, editor of this series, for her encouragement to write this book and for her helpful comments and feedback.

I have learned a lot about the impact of childhood eczema from the families who kindly agreed to participate in interviews for my PhD. I am very grateful to them for telling me about their experiences of caring for their children. In addition, after I had started my research on skin conditions, my oldest son developed severe eczema while he was a baby. My own personal experience of caring for him has helped me to understand the impact of eczema on young children and their families.

The names and other identifying details in all the case material and quotations in this book have been altered in order to protect the identity of those involved.

What is eczema?

"When he was first born he had beautiful skin, really soft ... but he turned three months and he just came out in this rash. I took him to the doctors and I had a feeling it was, and he said it's infantile eczema and it will go by the time he's a year old, but it didn't go, it got worse."

"She was about four months old when it first appeared. I went to the GP. I guessed it was eczema."

"I took him to the doctors and they said it was eczema ... I breast-fed him for one year and you would have thought that breast-feeding a baby it would be protected. So I think I felt a bit cheated actually."

This book is about the type of eczema known as 'atopic eczema'. This is the type of eczema with which people are most familiar. It is an itchy skin condition, which is most common in childhood and which often occurs on hands and in the creases behind the knees and elbows. It varies a lot in severity and can affect just one or two small areas of the body or it can be very extensive and cover nearly all the skin.

The appearance of skin affected by eczema can vary. Often the skin appears reddened and it can become thickened over time, particularly when it has been scratched a lot. It can also appear dry and flaky, with marked skin creases. When the eczema is infected, it often appears 'weepy' and has a 'crust' on it. Sometimes it looks more like a raised bumpy rash, and in children from an Afro-Caribbean background the skin can appear much darker where it is affected by eczema.

The word eczema actually comes from the Greek and means 'to boil out'. The word 'dermatitis' (which means 'inflamed skin') is sometimes used instead of eczema. So 'atopic dermatitis' is the same as 'atopic eczema'. 'Atopic' is another confusing word that literally means 'alien' and refers to a tendency to develop asthma, eczema and hayfever that runs through families. So 'atopic eczema' is the type of eczema that is strongly associated with these other conditions and which often does run in families.

There are in fact other types of eczema, such as seborrhoeic eczema or nummular eczema or contact dermatitis. These are less common than atopic eczema and require different approaches to treatment, so it is important to be clear about which type of eczema we are referring to. Throughout this book, whenever the word eczema is used, it is atopic eczema that is being referred to.

The British Association of Dermatologists has recently published diagnostic criteria for atopic eczema which help clarify the cluster of symptoms which make up this condition. It is important to remember that there is no simple 'test' to diagnose atopic eczema and that the diagnosis is made by identifying this cluster of familiar symptoms. In the past there has been a lot of variation in the diagnosis of atopic eczema and these guidelines help to ensure that everyone is using the same criteria for the diagnosis.

Box 1. Diagnostic guidelines for atopic eczema.

Must have:
An itchy skin condition
Plus three or more of the following:

(1) History of involvement of the skin creases such as folds of the elbows, behind the knees, fronts of the ankles or around the neck (including the cheeks in young children).

(2) A personal history of asthma or hayfever (or history of atopic disease in a first-degree relative in children under 4).

(3) A history of general dry skin in the last year.

(4) Visible flexural eczema (or eczema involving the cheeks/forehead and outer limbs in children under 4).

(5) Onset in the first 2 years of life.

How common is eczema?

Atopic eczema is most common during childhood and the rates do decrease with age. It is hard to give exact figures because of the differences between the age groups and because of differences in the criteria used for defining eczema. Between 10 and 15 per cent of children under seven develop eczema whereas only 2 per cent of 12–15-year-olds have eczema. This is an encouraging statistic because it does mean that most children do grow out of it. Unfortunately we are not yet able to tell which these children will be. So when your doctor tells you that it is likely that your child will grow out of it, this is true for this group of children overall, but you unfortunately have to wait and see for our own child.

Rates of eczema are different in different ethnic groups. For example, for reasons we don't fully understand, rates of eczema are higher among children from Afro-Caribbean backgrounds born in London. This can be particularly frustrating for families who find that their child's skin condition also improves when they return to a Caribbean climate, for example on holiday.

Why is eczema more common in younger children?

We don't really have a good answer for why eczema affects children mostly when they are young. It does suggest that it might be linked in some way to maturation or establishing biological processes.

This often means that your child is worst affected by eczema while still a baby, toddler or pre-schooler. In some ways this is very fortunate, because young children are less self-conscious and they are less likely to become embarrassed by their eczema. However, it also means that you have to manage all the normal developmental processes that occur in this age group as well as managing the eczema treatment. Temper tantrums, difficulties with sleeping and eating problems are all very common in this age group. Language and cognitive skills are all still developing and it is much harder to reason and negotiate with a 2- or 3-year-old than a 9-year-old.

The fact that eczema is at its worst during this time is part of what makes it so difficult to manage eczema in childhood. Your child is going through all the developmental stages that are part of becoming more independent and ready for life outside the home, including school. The sorts of difficulties that are very common in this age group are often exacerbated by the presence of eczema.

Why is eczema becoming more common?

We know now that eczema has become more common over the past 20 years. Although many people originally thought this was just because it was diagnosed or treated more, we now know that the rates really are on the increase along with the rates of allergy and asthma. Although there are no definite answers as to why this is happening, there are some theories. Some people believe it is due to the reduction in the exposure of children to 'normal' infections or illnesses. The theory is that it is by fighting these 'normal' bugs that our immune systems become fully activated. It is argued that this process has become disrupted by our living protected lives. Our bodies then become 'over-sensitive' to harmless bugs or environmental agents and this results in an increase in atopic conditions.

Another theory it that it is related to other changes in the way we live, for example living in centrally heated houses with reduced air circulation due to double glazing, with a lot of soft furnishing and carpets. These sorts of environments lead to a increased numbers of house dust mites and this may contribute to the increase in rates of childhood eczema.

Other possible explanations include the increase in air pollutants and other environment changes due to increased industrialisation. For some reason it appears that the increase in rates of eczema is most marked in the more afflu-ent areas of the world, which does suggest it is related to changes in our lifestyles.

What causes eczema?

Unfortunately there is no simple answer to this. Even dermatologists can have heated debates about the role of different factors in causing eczema. Some relevant factors are now well established by research. For example, it is clearly established that eczema runs in families and hence genetic factors are important. Others are more controversial. These include the link between allergy and eczema, and the role of diet.

It is also important to remember the difference between true *causes* of eczema and factors that are important in *maintaining* the eczema. Once eczema has become established, the skin becomes much more sensitive and substances that would not normally cause a problem to healthy skin do exacerbate the symptoms of eczema. Several substances fall into this category, for example wool fibres, dog hairs, chemicals in washing powder and some preservatives in creams. Because the skin affected by eczema is dry and cracked, it is much easier for irritant substances to cross the skin boundary and cause irritation. Rather than providing a firm 'wall' which prevents substances leaking into or out of the body, skin affected by eczema is weakened or leaky. Substances that would not normally cause irritation are able to get into the skin and then they do cause a problem.

Although eczema and the other atopic conditions do tend to run in families, this is not in a completely predictable way, so it is not possible to say that any particular family will definitely have a child with an atopic condition. If you or your partner have a strong family history of eczema or asthma then you are more likely to have a child with one or both of these conditions. So there is definitely a genetic component to atopic conditions but this does not enable us to predict the condition for any one individual.

Is eczema caused by allergy?

This is a controversial area at the moment, and causes a lot of confusion and debate. Before we start, it is best to be clear by what is meant by allergy. An allergic reaction is the consequence of the body's 'overreaction' to a harmless substance. The body detects what it considers a 'foreign' substance and mistakenly interprets it as dangerous. This activates the immune system and sets off a chemical response in the body and leads to a raised level of immunoglobulin E (IgE) in the body. A true allergy is therefore very different from the type of irritation caused in skin affected by eczema by a substance such as wool or soap as described in the section above. Food is usually thought of as the main allergen related to eczema but other types of allergen, such as house dust mite, may be relevant.

In some children it is easy to demonstrate an allergic reaction. For example, some children develop an immediate skin reaction, known as 'urticaria' within minutes of being in contact with what is normally considered a harmless substance, such as egg or cow's milk. Urticaria looks like nettle rash and is often very itchy and uncomfortable. Although these types of allergies are rare, they are very easily identified and treatment involves avoidance of the food trigger.

There is also a very dangerous form of allergy known as anaphylaxis, which is again easy to identify and usually the cause can be found. An anaphylactic reaction causes swelling in the mouth and tongue, difficulty with breathing and widespread urticaria. This can lead to collapse and even death due to the swelling in the windpipe. For reasons we do not yet fully understand, this type of reaction is often associated with peanuts or other nuts and has increased in prevalence over the past 20 years. Although very serious and frightening, it is usually possible to identify the cause of this sort of a reaction and avoid the trigger substance.

But most allergies are not so easily identified and the vagueness of the symptoms described, as well as the difficulties testing for allergies, means that it is very hard to establish the cause of many reported 'allergies'. In addition, sometimes an allergic reaction may not occur immediately and may be delayed for several hours, so this makes it particularly hard to identify the allergen. So, although many people do think that their eczema is caused by an allergy, this can be very hard to prove.

Although there are some types of laboratory tests which can be used for detecting allergies, these are not very reliable. They may sometimes appear to indicate a high level of allergy, when in fact the person has no significant symptoms of an allergy when they come in contact with the allergen, or, vice versa, they sometimes indicate a low level of allergy when someone has very marked symptoms when they do eat the food or come in contact with the allergen. For this reason, many doctors are reluctant to suggest using these types of tests because they often make the situation less clear, rather than helping to clarify the presence of an allergy.

There has been a huge increase in the awareness of allergies in the past 10 years and allergy testing has become quite an industry. Many doctors do feel suspicious of some allergy clinics because at the moment there is very little strong evidence to back up some of the claims made. It is important to be aware of this because it is too easy to clutch at straws when you feel that no cure is being offered.

On the other hand, a small proportion of children with eczema do have a true allergy and it is important not to deny this just because there is an overemphasis on allergies in general. Estimates vary, but some experts think that food allergy may be an important cause of eczema in up to 10 per cent of young children affected by eczema. A slightly higher proportion of children may find that an allergen is a contributing factor for their eczema, although it is not the main cause of the eczema.

Is eczema caused by stress?

As a society we are becoming more aware of the link between the body and the mind, and we recognise now that psychological factors, such as stress, are important in our understanding of how illnesses affect us.

Unlike in many other illnesses, the link between the mind and the body has been seen as relevant for eczema for many years. Indeed there has even been an assumption that eczema is a 'psychosomatic' illness, in other words an illness that is caused by psychological factors rather than physical or organic ones. This probably resulted from several factors. There is no doubt that many people with eczema can identify episodes when their eczema gets worse which are directly linked to stressful periods in their lives. In these situations it does appear that the stress has 'caused' the eczema. There is also no doubt that eczema and the discomfort it brings can cause a high level of stress itself. Hence we get a 'chicken and egg' problem. Did the eczema cause the stress or did the stress cause the eczema, or is it a bit of both?

Another reason why eczema has been labelled a psychosomatic illness is because we have never had a very convincing medical explanation of what causes eczema and what causes flares in the condition. When no physical cause can be found for a condition, it has often been assumed that the cause must then be psychological. This assumption is also common in other conditions where the physical cause is not well understood. Gradually, as our understanding of the physical cause becomes more sophisticated we realise that what we previously called psychosomatic illnesses are sometimes physical illnesses that were just poorly understood at the time.

The reality is that with a condition like eczema it is often hard to separate out the biological and the psychological factors. The cause and effect works in both directions and each influences the other. We should keep an open mind and be aware that stressful situations may well make eczema worse, but that it would be misleading to say that eczema can be caused by stress alone. However, when we are very stressed we find it harder to cope with the difficulties presented by eczema, such as managing the treatment and tolerating the symptoms. So most people also find they are less well able to manage the treatment regime when they are more stressed and probably do it less effectively, hence making it more likely the symptoms will get worse.

CASE STUDY CASE STUDY CASE STUDY CASE STUDY

David

David was born after a normal pregnancy and birth. He was born two weeks after his expected date and his mother noticed he appeared to have quite dry skin. At about four months of age he began to develop a raised itchy rash on his cheeks, forehead and tummy. He had great difficulty sleeping and his mother would frequently find him rubbing his face against the cot bumper. He was diagnosed as having eczema by his GP and prescribed emollients and bath oil.

David's mother frequently tried to identify the cause of his eczema. She went through phases of thinking it was due to what David ate, the washing powder she used, the central heating system and the hard water in their area. None of these factors appeared to be the only cause of his symptoms and David's mother was unable to identify one single cause. In the end, she attributed David's eczema to 'bad luck' and something he had been born with. Although David's mother had never had eczema, her partner did have eczema throughout his childhood and his mother (David's grandmother) remembered it had followed a similar pattern to David's eczema.

As David got older, the distribution of his eczema changed. It got a lot better on his face but affected his hands and backs of his knees. It remained very similar until he was about four when it gradually began to improve and although David continued to have quite dry skin, the eczema itself resolved by the time he was eight.

Summary

- Atopic eczema is a common condition in childhood which often improves as the child grows older.

- It has become more common over the past 20 years.

- The causes of eczema are not fully understood but it is known to be a hereditary condition.

- Although allergy may be an important cause for a small minority of young children, it is usually not the main cause of eczema.

- Eczema is often associated with stress, but it is likely that the symptoms of eczema cause stress, as well as the stress making the eczema worse.

What is the best treatment for eczema?

"I'm just worried of the long-term effects on them of having these steroid creams. I know obviously its sort of a toss-up between having sore skin now or having problems later. I know there is no easy solution but I think sometimes I'd be happier trying to find out what causes it as opposed to just continually treating the symptoms.**"**

"He doesn't like putting his creams on, he hates the wet wraps. He's very hard work and it's constant. You've got to keep on at him.**"**

"Also if you take him out and he's scratching people do stare. And people are always saying, 'Have you tried this', and 'Have you taken him to the doctor?', 'Have you done that?' And sometimes I think, oh, just smile and say yes.**"**

It can be surprisingly hard to find the best treatment for your child's eczema. This is partly because of the nature of eczema itself. Eczema varies such a lot over time and sometimes appears to get better or worse for no apparent reason, so it can be hard to work out whether the changes you see in your child's skin are related to changes you have made in the treatment you are using. In addition, even with the best possible treatment the eczema may not disappear – it should become more manageable and may gradually decrease in severity, but for many children it is a chronic condition and so it may be unrealistic to expect that a total cure is possible.

But it is also hard to find the best treatment because of conflicting information about what treatments are most effective. There is the established, conventional medical treatment that involves using emollients to moisturise the skin, avoiding irritants such as soap or wool fibres, steroid cream to control flare-ups or severe patches of eczema and antibiotics if the eczema becomes infected. However, many families worry about the long-term effects of using steroid creams and would prefer to find the 'cause' of flares rather than treating the symptoms. There are also many different types of complementary therapy which suggest alternative ways of managing eczema, and it can be hard to find out exactly how effective these are.

In addition to the difficulties in finding the best treatment plan, there is then the difficult task of actually carrying out the treatment effectively. The conventional treatment for eczema is in principle very simple. However, it is surprisingly hard to carry out with a young child who may be physically uncomfortable, and who may experience the treatment as tedious (at best) and even painful (at worst). There are good reasons why the treatment may not be as effective as you hoped, simply because it is hard to stick consistently to the treatment regime over a long period of time.

You will probably get much conflicting advice about managing childhood eczema. This chapter explains how to make sense of this advice and describes how frustratingly little clear evidence there is. This chapter then goes on to look at how to overcome some of the difficulties in using the treatment effectively.

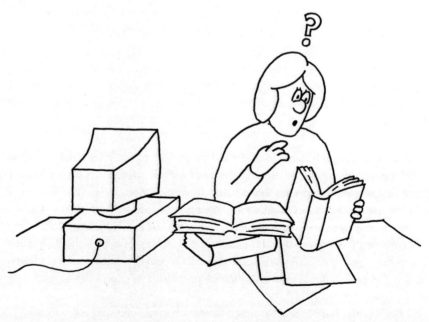

It can be hard to make sense of all the conflicting advice you get about how to manage your child's eczema.

How do I know what treatment to use?

The answer to this may seem obvious: you rely on the best advice you can get. However, with a child with eczema you may find that you are given lots of different and sometimes conflicting advice, and it is hard to know who or what to believe. Your GP will advise you about the conventional method of treating eczema using emollients (moisturisers) and, if necessary, steroids. However, eczema is a common condition and it is often the case that friends, relatives and even strangers will offer you advice based on their own experience. In addition, you are likely to come across advertisements for complementary or 'alternative' treatments for eczema, such as herbal medicines or homeopathic remedies. It is difficult to weigh up all the different types of advice you are given to work out how best to treat your child.

Within the medical world it is usually accepted that the only way of proving that a treatment is effective is to carry out a 'randomised controlled trial'. This involves comparing the new treatment with another treatment that appears very similar to the one being tested but which is known to have no significant effect (a placebo) or comparing the new treatment with the existing best type of treatment. In order to make sure that any observed improvement is due to the actual treatment used rather than just to chance, you have to test the new treatment on a large number of people. Rather than allowing people to choose the treatment they would prefer, the people have to be allocated to one of the treatments in a random way to avoid any bias. Finally, you have to make sure that neither the people taking part in the trial nor the doctors looking at the results are able to work out which is the active treatment and which is the placebo – otherwise they may (consciously or unconsciously) try to ensure that they get the result they want.

Given all these demands on what counts as 'proof' for an effective treatment, it is perhaps not surprising that there are relatively few of these types of studies that have been carried out on treatments for childhood eczema. In addition, when a treatment has become widely accepted through clinical practice, it often then makes it hard to carry out a trial because it would not be justifiable to withhold a treatment that is widely believed to be effective, such as an emollient. Many of the trials that have been done are also rather artificial; for example, they only evaluate treatment over a few weeks, and yet eczema is a chronic condition and so it would make sense to look at how effective a treatment is in the long term. There has been a review (Hoare *et al.*, 2000) of all the different treatment trials for eczema and this illustrates how much of the current standard treatment for eczema is not based on strict 'proof' as outlined above (see 'Recommended further reading' for the publication details of this report).

So, as is the case in a lot of other areas of medicine, the treatment currently recommended relies a lot on clinical experience rather than on highly rigorous scientific 'proof'. Clinical experience is nonetheless an extremely valuable tool.

A doctor who has seen several hundred children with eczema is likely to have learned some very useful things from that experience. But the reliance on clinical judgement does help explain why you end up with conflicting advice. So you therefore have to make a judgement about the likely quality of the advice you are being given. For example, a dermatologist will have the advantage of having access to recent specialist studies as well as his or her clinical experience, and he or she is more likely to have dealt with severe or difficult-to-treat eczema. Your GP will have seen lots of children with mild or moderate eczema, but he or she is not a specialist in this specific area and is unlikely to have the same depth of knowledge as a dermatologist. Your friend or the 'helpful' stranger who stops you to give you advice may well have a bit of useful personal experience, but it is likely to be based on one example, or at best a handful of examples, and whilst it may be given with the best of intentions it is likely to be of limited help.

Which conventional treatments have been shown to be effective for eczema?

Emollients

Ironically, there are very few research trials proving the effectiveness of emollients (moisturisers) and yet these are almost universally recommended for eczema and nearly everybody accepts they are effective. This is partly because they are so widely accepted as an effective treatment that there is little need to prove any benefit and because there are so few disadvantages to using emollients. So there has never been much of a need to test whether or not emollients are effective or not. Unfortunately, one consequence of this is that there is therefore no evidence to support one type of emollient over another, so the best type of emollient to use is probably the one the child or family prefer and the one they will use most effectively.

Steroids

Topical steroids have been shown to be effective in controlling the symptoms of eczema in clinical trials but again there is little evidence to help choose between different formulations. (Topical means that they are applied directly to the skin.) There is very little research on what is the most effective way of using steroids, for example is it best to apply them once or twice a day? Is it best to use a mild steroid more frequently or a stronger steroid less frequently? This problem is gradually being addressed and there has been one recent study comparing using a mild steroid frequently, with using a more potent steroid in short bursts. However, these sorts of studies which more closely resemble 'real life' are few and far between and would be very helpful in answering some of the questions around how to use steroids in safe way.

Many parents worry about the side effects of using steroids. There is no doubt that the stronger steroid creams can cause problems if used over the long term, particularly when applied to delicate skin such as the face. However, the current recommendations for how to use steroids effectively and safely do now take this into account. See the section below (p. 20) on how to use conventional treatments effectively for details of how to make appropriate use of steroids.

Tacrolimus

There is now good evidence of the effectiveness of a new treatment, known as tacrolimus, when it is compared with a placebo treatment or topical steroids. Tacrolimus is a cream that has an immunosuppressant action. It is thought that tacrolimus may be very helpful for treating moderate to severe eczema instead of steroids, and it has been shown to be more effective than a weak topical steroid cream in research studies. The attraction of tacrolimus for many people is that is does not appear to have serious long-term side effects, such as the skin thinning that occurs with potent steroids, and could be an alternative for people who are specifically concerned about this aspect of steroids. Nonetheless it is relatively new, and so it is hard to know yet how useful it will prove to be in the long-term management of eczema. Some children do experience a burning sensation when the cream is applied at first but this side effect does not appear to be harmful and does appear to reduce over time.

Eradication of house dust mites

Eradicating house dust mites has been found to be of some use in controlling eczema in some studies. However, reducing house dust mites is a particularly difficult task and what the studies have not yet addressed is how useful this form of treatment is in real life over the long term. It is an extremely time-consuming task to try and reduce house dust mites and involves regular vacuum cleaning, damp dusting and keeping soft furnishing to a minimum. It can also be very expensive to replace existing carpets or soft furnishing with more suitable ones. Only a few families are able to sustain this type of approach in the long term, and so this may make this type of approach of limited use for chronic eczema. For children with both asthma and eczema it is probably worth taking simple measures to keep the number of dust mites restricted. For example, if you are replacing carpets, it is better to have a wooden floor or vinyl rather than thick carpets in your child's bedroom. It is also worth 'damp dusting' rather than dusting with polish because this is a more effective way of picking up dust.

Other specialised treatments

There are other very specialised treatments for severe, chronic eczema such as PUVA (a type of light therapy combined with an oral drug called psoralen) and cyclosporin (an immunosuppressant medication). However, these are only usually offered to older children who have very severe chronic eczema that has not improved over time.

What is the evidence supporting 'complementary therapies' as effective treatments for eczema?

There are a growing number of 'complementary therapies' for eczema, as well as for other medical conditions. These include homeopathy, acupuncture, Chinese herbal medicine and aromatherapy. However, this area is a bit of a minefield – it is hard to make sense of what is claimed for these treatments because the type of evidence which the medical world considers valuable is very scarce. Instead, you have to rely on the practitioner him or herself and anecdotal evidence. Nonetheless, there is no doubt that some people have found complementary approaches helpful and a very large number of people will try a form of complementary medicine for their child's eczema, even if they are a bit sceptical, because they feel they have nothing to lose and continue to hope that there must be a successful treatment somewhere.

There are many other indirect benefits of consulting a complementary therapist. All these approaches do emphasise the importance of seeing the child and family in a holistic way rather than just concentrating on symptoms. Many families like this sort of approach because unfortunately they will probably only have had relatively brief meetings with either their GP or dermatologist because of the short time available in a typical NHS service. It can be extremely useful to talk through your concerns about your child and his or her eczema, and this type of consultation may be very helpful irrespective of whether or not the treatment itself works.

Chinese herbal treatment

There are some carefully carried out trials of Chinese herbal treatment for eczema that were properly randomised and controlled and hence 'scientifically respectable'. The first two studies did demonstrate that the Chinese herbal treatment was significantly more effective than a placebo treatment. However, two subsequent studies have not found this benefit, which makes it hard to interpret the findings until more studies are carried out. There are some potentially very dangerous side effects of some Chinese herbal treatments and these have caused a high level of concern about the use of these treatments. In addition many children find them so unpleasant to take that they are unable to use the treatment as prescribed.

Massage

There is also a small amount of research evidence supporting the use of massage therapy with young children. In one study mothers of young children were taught massage techniques to use on their child in addition to their standard treatment package for eczema and some benefits were found, including an improvement in coping and a reduction in anxiety.

Acupuncture and homeopathy

There have been positive clinical reports for both acupuncture and homeopathy, and both of these are sometimes available on the NHS. However, there are no formal treatment trials for childhood eczema that have been reported in the literature. It is therefore very important for these treatments to be evaluated systematically in the near future. If they are effective, then they should be made available more widely. However, if they are not effective, it is important that the resources of either the individual family, or of the NHS as a service, are not inappropriately used.

Evening primrose oil

There have been some trials that do show that evening primrose oil may improve the symptoms of eczema. However, the newer and larger studies have failed to find an improvement. So at the moment it seems unlikely that evening primrose oil will become a very successful treatment. On the other hand it may turn out to be of benefit to a small minority of people, and the advantages are that it is unlikely to be harmful.

When is it appropriate to try complementary therapies?

So, if you can't use research evidence to back up your decision, how should you decide whether or not to try a complementary therapy? Your decision should be based firstly on ensuring you choose a properly trained and experienced therapist who is a member of a professional body. Although this does not guarantee that their treatment will work, it does provide some reassurance that they are properly qualified and the treatment will be safe.

The Royal College of Nursing recommends asking the following questions to help you evaluate whether you should pursue treatment with a complementary therapist:

- What are your qualifications and how long was the training?
- Are you a member of a recognised professional body?
- Will you keep my GP informed of treatment I receive?

- Are you insured against accident negligence and malpractice?
- Are the records you keep on patients confidential?
- Have you had previous experience of treating eczema successfully?
- What is the cost of the treatment?
- How many sessions will I need?

Then it is important to consider how happy you are with the answers given.

- Did the practitioner answer your questions clearly and to your satisfaction?
- Were you provided with any background in writing on the therapy or the clinic?
- Did they provide evidence of their qualification or contact details for their professional body?
- Did you feel that the practitioner conducted themselves in a professional manner?
- Did the practitioner make excessive claims for their treatment? Be wary if they promise to be able to cure eczema completely.

These guidelines will help you to make an informed choice about whether the type of complementary treatment you have chosen is worth trying.

Do dietary treatments for eczema work?

This is again another controversial area in this field with too few good studies that would enable us to answer this question definitively. Restricted diets during pregnancy and while breastfeeding have been used to try and prevent eczema developing. In addition, diets have also been used after eczema has developed to try and improve symptoms.

There is some evidence that dietary restrictions do have some effect for a small minority of young children with eczema. However, there are real difficulties in using these dietary restrictions effectively, and many people are wary of advising the use of restricted diets because of the possible complications of restricting any young child's food intake. A fuller discussion of the use of restricted diets for treating eczema is covered in Chapter 6.

Getting the best from your treatment: how to use the conventional treatments as effectively as possible

How should I use emollients?

The key to using emollients effectively is to apply them regularly to prevent your child's skin from drying out. Cracked and broken skin affected by eczema allows moisture to evaporate from the skin and emollients help to provide an oily layer that will trap moisture inside. Broken or cracked skin is also a less effective barrier and will make it easier for infections to grow. It is also helpful to add bath oils to your child's bath water and avoid the use of soap or bubble bath which dry out the skin. Your aim is to keep the skin constantly moisturised, rather than allowing it to dry out between treatments.

Emollients come in different forms: lotions, creams and ointments. Whilst lotions and creams are easier to put on and feel less greasy, they contain higher amounts of water and need to be applied more frequently. Ointments are very greasy and help retain moisture well but many children find them unpleasant because they feel heavy and sticky on their skin. The most important choice is not about which particular brand of emollient to use, or whether to use a cream or ointment, but which type will be most effective for your child. Even if an ointment is better in theory, if your child is reluctant to use it or refuses to let you put it on properly, it will not be effective. If your child feels more comfortable using a cream, and practically, you are able to apply it frequently, then this may be more effective in practice than an ointment.

There is a real lack of good research on the different forms of emollients, despite the fact that they are almost universally recommended for eczema. There are at least 30 different emollients which your GP or dermatologist can choose to prescribe for your child, and a vast number of other products available over the counter or from specialist shops such as health shops. In addition, there are 10 different bath preparations which can be prescribed. Yet there is no good evidence from research to indicate whether any of these different preparations are significantly better or worse than any other. So the choice in the end will largely be down to you and the experience of whoever is prescribing the emollient.

The ideal situation is for you to be able to try out different types yourself to find the one that suits your child. It can be difficult to persuade your doctor to keep letting you try different ones, but it is worth it in the long run. In addition, be careful not to jump to conclusions – remember how much eczema varies and allow a sufficient amount of time before you conclude that a particular type is or is not effective. Occasionally a child may react to the perfume or preservatives in an emollient and it can be hard to identify these. If in doubt, try comparing using one emollient on one part of the body (e.g. an arm) and a different one on another. If there is a significant problem due to a specific perfume or preservative, this should help make it more obvious.

My child hates having her cream put on so we often end up with both of us cross – what can I do to make it an easier time for us both?

Your aim is to keep the skin soft and moisturised and this means applying moisturiser regularly in order to prevent the skin drying out. This is time-consuming and for many parents and children it can become a battleground. Children vary a lot in how they react to having moisturisers applied. It is possible for this to be a very soothing experience for a child and certainly it can feel very pleasant, like a massage. However, if the child's skin is already itchy and uncomfortable, then undressing to apply the cream and the actual contact of the cream on the skin can feel uncomfortable and actually lead to scratching as the cream is applied, or just after.

Also, like all of us, children have good days and bad days – there are almost certain to be times when they are reluctant to have their cream put on. Remember that treating eczema may involve thousands of occasions on which you have to apply moisturiser. Even if you only do it three times a day, that is more than one thousand times over one whole year. It is not easy for anyone to keep up their motivation and their child's cooperation over all these repeated episodes.

It is helpful to consider whether this is a problem that is only related to eczema treatment or whether these sort of battles occur regularly during the day over other routine tasks, such as tidying up toys, or doing something that you need them to do, like eat lunch. There is a huge variation in the amount of oppositional behaviour children show at different ages, as well as a lot of variation between children. Some children will only throw a handful of real tantrums a year, whereas others will regularly have tantrums many times in one day. In addition, whilst it is relatively normal for a 2-year-old to have regular tantrums, these should begin to reduce by the time they are 4 years old.

So, is this a problem that is affecting lots of areas of your child's life and/or which is unexpected for this age group, or is it just the eczema treatment that causes the problems? If it is the first of these, you need to think about using the general strategies that are helpful for managing any young child's behaviour. There are some very helpful books about managing the behaviour of young children – see 'Recommended further reading' at the back of the book. There are also some suggestions for managing difficult behaviour in Chapter 3.

If the problem is mostly restricted to applying emollients then there may be something you can do to change your management of your child's skin routine to improve the situation.

Improving your skin care routine

The general principles are to think long-term and to plan ahead how you are going to manage, given that this treatment has to be done so regularly. There are practical things you can do to make life more bearable if your child dislikes having the emollients applied. None of these techniques will work forever, but they may refresh your routine for a while. You cannot expect any young child to meekly sit through thousands of treatment sessions without showing signs of boredom or irritability. Nor can you expect them to accept the logic that it is important to apply creams regularly to keep their skin supple and moisturised. What you can do is minimise the distress they experience and the restriction they feel because of the routine. You can also try and prevent this becoming a regular battle between the two of you by dealing with your own frustration so that you can manage your child's difficulties as calmly and positively as possible.

However, all of these suggestions can be difficult to carry out when you yourself are worn out and fed up with the routine. It may be difficult for you to think positively about the skin-care routine if you are already at this stage. You may need to consider arranging some extra help to get you to a stage when you can begin to think positively again. Although it is never easy to find someone who can substitute for you in caring for your child, you may be able to find someone to do the other chores for which you can be replaced more easily, such as cleaning or shopping. Even a short break for yourself can help you to recharge your batteries and to feel that you are able to continue to give your child the care he or she needs. Looking after a child with chronic eczema does involve a large burden of care and you should not feel guilty about building into your plan times for you to get a break.

HELPFUL TIPS! HELPFUL TIPS! HELPFUL TIPS! HELPFUL

- Make the whole situation more comfortable: have plenty of distractions available. For a very young baby or child, novelty is very effective and there are lots of ordinary objects that are novel and interesting to your toddler or child, e.g. shiny or scrunchy objects, that look, feel or sound different. Give these to your child **before** they become uncomfortable rather than once they are already itching or scratching. For toddlers or older children, watching cartoons or interesting TV programmes or listening to tapes of fun songs can provide useful distraction. So set up the situation in advance to help make it more bearable.

- If possible allow your child some choice and control over the routine. Allow them to do some patting in of cream, let them choose which tape they want to have on while you do the cream. Let them choose what toys they want to bring in with them while you put the cream on.

- Keep the emollient handy so that you can apply it at times when the child is relatively settled: be proactive, and seize opportunities when you can. It doesn't matter if it's half an hour or so before you planned to put the cream on. Catch them while you can.

- Invest some time in finding the best treatment for your child's skin. There are many different emollients available on prescription. Ideally you should have the opportunity to try out different ones in order to choose the best one for you and your child. The different products contain different preservatives and perfumes and it is possible that your child may be sensitive to the added ingredients in the emollient. Alternatively, they may prefer the fun of dispensers rather than tubes or pots.

- Think about how to manage your own reaction as well as your child's reaction. If you become cross very easily, or if you become very upset when carrying out the treatment, then it may be that it is you that has the difficulty with the treatment rather than your child. This is not 'your fault' because there is certainly a reason why it upsets you or makes you angry – you do not feel these emotions out of choice! However, having some time talking through why you find it frustrating, preferably with someone who does understand about eczema, such as a specialist nurse or another mother, may help to reduce the tension a bit. It is important to realise that this treatment is not easy for anyone to carry out all the time and everyone does find it difficult at times.

How safe are steroid creams for treating eczema?

If your child has mild eczema, you may be able to control the eczema using only emollients. However, if he or she has patches of severe eczema or has a flare-up causing an exacerbation of his or her eczema, you will probably be advised to use steroid creams. Many parents are very wary of using steroids – sometimes for good reasons; sometimes because of unnecessary fears. Dermatologists have started using the phrase 'steroid phobia' because of the widespread suspicion about the long-term use of steroids, which they feel is unjustified. So how safe are steroids and what is the best way of using them safely?

Steroids were first developed in the 1950s. At first, they were greeted enthusiastically and it was hoped that they would provide an effective treatment for many conditions, including eczema. In the early days, even the most potent forms would have been used on all parts of the body, even the face. Gradually, the negative side effects of steroids became more apparent. There are many mothers of children with eczema today who were treated with strong steroids as a child, and have the consequent skin thinning which understandably makes them more suspicious of using steroids on their own children. Also, steroids that are absorbed into the bloodstream can have an effect on growth, and this is a serious side effect for children.

Steroids, like emollients, come in many different forms and again your doctor has the choice of a large number of different brands or types to choose from. The most important feature he or she will take into account is the strength of the steroid. Steroids are graded in a standardised way from 'mild' to 'very potent' and it is very important to be clear which type you are using for your child. Even now, when surveys are carried out, many parents are not clear about the strength of the steroid they are currently using on their child. This is not helped by the extremely confusing names and labelling of products, and the number of products available, which makes it hard to keep up with all the brands. The general rule of prescribing is to use the lowest strength that is effective in controlling the symptoms, because the higher the level of potency the higher the risk of side effects. Also, to reduce rebound effects, it is important to gradually reduce the potency rather than abruptly stop a potent or very potent treatment.

The other widespread concern about steroids is that they are 'just suppressing' the symptoms of the eczema rather than 'curing' it. Many families describe how the eczema reappears immediately when the steroid treatment is stopped and that this makes them feel that it cannot be the most appropriate treatment available. The problem with this is that it presupposes that there is a 'cure' out there if only you could find it. However, most families find that they spend a long time looking for this cure and it rarely, if ever, materialises. If you have tried all the obvious 'cures' and accept that there is no 'cure' waiting to be found, this helps with this dilemma. Although it is true that steroid creams may only be suppressing the symptoms, this may be worthwhile in itself and may lead to a much better quality of life. Also, if there are no other alternatives, then the benefits of steroids may well outweigh the disadvantages. So the crucial decision is deciding whether the advantages outweigh the possibility of side effects.

One of the problems with weighing up the disadvantages against the advantages of using steroids is that there is a lack of good research on steroid use which would provide guidance in the long term for the way that steroids are used in real life. There are good studies that suggest that steroids are effective when compared to placebos, but there are few studies suggesting which particular preparations are the most effective or the most effective way to use them. The controlled studies that have been carried out to examine the adverse effects of steroid use have typically been quite short-term and hence do not provide much useful information when many children are affected by eczema for several years rather than weeks or months.

HELPFUL TIPS! HELPFUL TIPS! HELPFUL TIPS! HELPFUL

There are now very clear recommendations about the use of steroids and these should be followed carefully to reduce the risk of side effects.

- Apply the steroid sparingly, just a thin layer is needed. There are three ways to help guide you in judging how much to apply. One method involves measuring the amount of steroid used in terms

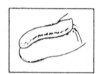

One adult *Fingertip Unit* (FTU)

The diagrams of the child (below) show how many adult *Fingertip Units* of cream or ointment are required to cover each area of the child's body.

	Face & Neck	Arm & Hand	Leg & Foot	Trunk (Front)	Trunk (Back) inc. Buttocks
Age	Number of FTUs				
3-6 mth	1	1	1½	1	1½
1-2 y	1½	1½	2	2	3
3-5 y	1½	2	3	3	3½
6-10 y	2	2½	4½	3½	5

Figure 1. A parent's guide to the use of topical treatment. Reproduced from Long, C.C., Mills, C.M. and Finlay A.Y. (1998) A parents' guide to the use of topical treatments, in 'A practical guide to topical therapy in children', *British Journal of Dermatology, 138,* 293-296. Reproduced by permission of Blackwell Publishing Ltd.

of 'fingertip units' (FTUs). This is the amount of cream that covers the length of an adult's last joint of their index finger. A very helpful chart is produced to show how much can be used for young children for different areas of their body. The disadvantage of this method is that it is hard to judge how much to use when only a small amount of the body area indicated is affected by eczema. After all it is common that only a small area of an arm will need treating with steroid, so how much of a unit should you use then?

- The second method involves estimating how many 'hand areas' are affected by eczema. A 'hand area' is the area made by the flat of your hand when your fingers are together. In other words if you put your hand palm down onto a surface with your fingers closed together, a 'hand area' is the area you are covering. One FTU will cover two hand areas, two FTUs will cover four hand areas, etc. This is helpful for estimating the amount of steroid needed for smaller areas of the body.

- The other method of judging how much to use is to apply only enough to give the skin a sheen or make it glisten slightly. Although this is still rather vague as well, it does emphasise the use of the smallest amount possible.

- Some doctors and nurses now also advise that emollients should be applied before the steroid cream, preferably at least 30 minutes before. This also seems to help reduce the amount of steroid needed and hence reduce the likely long-term side effects.

- Use the lowest level of potency that is effective for the symptoms. If on a high level of potency, gradually reduce down the levels as the eczema comes under control.

- Remember that although there are risks associated with long-term use of steroids, these can be reduced by applying the steroids according to current guidelines. Remember also that the reduction in inflammation achieved by using steroids may ▶

enable you to get back into control and manage your child's eczema more effectively. In addition, if the child is scratching less, then the skin will be damaged less, allowing more healing to take place. In the long term, using a short burst of steroids may enable you to regain control of the eczema and manage with emollients most of the time.

Steroids have their use in the treatment of eczema, but it is worth working hard to control the symptoms as much as possible with emollients and to keep the use of steroids to the minimum possible to regain control.

If your child has very severe chronic eczema, some dermatologists do prescribe the use of oral steroids. With oral steroids, the risk of side effects is much increased, because more of the active treatment is absorbed into the body. Any child on oral steroids needs to be monitored very carefully because of the possible side effects. In addition they need to be on the treatment for the shortest time possible to be gradually weaned off the medication.

How does wet wrapping work and why is it effective?

Wet wrapping involves literally wrapping your child in wet bandages after having applied their emollients and, if necessary, steroid creams. It is often suggested as the next line of treatment if the usual management of emollients and steroids is not helping to control the eczema. Although there are no controlled trials to support the use of wet wraps, they have become part of the standard treatment approach for severe eczema in the UK.

Wet wrapping appears to work at several different levels. Firstly, it effectively prevents your child from scratching, because the skin is so well covered by bandages. Secondly, as the water evaporates from the bandages over time, it cools the skin, and this can be very soothing for itchy skin. It also helps to rehydrate the skin both directly and indirectly by enclosing the emollient and enabling it to work for much longer than it normally would. Finally, it appears to help the body absorb the steroids more effectively, allowing the steroid to penetrate deeper into the skin. However, wet wraps cannot be used when the skin is infected as this might make the infection worse because the germs can multiply easily in warm wet conditions.

Wet wraps can be quite time-consuming to put on and certainly require a lot of practice to apply easily. You would have to learn how to put them on and can be shown how to do this by a nurse or dermatologist. In addition the National Eczema Society produces a helpful guide to using wet wraps, including providing details of how to get hold of stickers, videos and story books specifically designed to encourage children in their use of wet wraps.

The main obstacle to using wet wraps is that they require quite a lot of time and effort on your part, as well as cooperation from your child. Some children, particularly if they can immediately see and feel the benefits of wet wrapping, do adapt to having the wraps put on relatively easily and, once you get used to putting them on, it just becomes part of the routine. However, for other children it is difficult to get them to keep still and cooperate, and this can be a very fraught time. You have to decide if the benefits outweigh the disadvantages.

HELPFUL TIPS! HELPFUL TIPS! HELPFUL TIPS! HELPFUL

- Get yourself well organised before starting, and enlist a 'helper' for the first few times to ensure you can get the bandages on within a reasonable length of time.

- Make the experience as positive as possible for your child, by involving them with some of the preparation and being very positive with them about their contribution. Distraction is also a useful technique, so you could watch a video together as you put the bandages on.

- It is worth choosing your time carefully. At the end of the day, tired young children rapidly lose their patience and it is always much harder when your child is tired and irritable. You may have to choose an earlier time to put the wet wraps on.

CASE STUDY CASE STUDY CASE STUDY CASE STUDY

Sarah

Sarah began to develop eczema when she was about 10 weeks old. At first she had dry itchy patches on her cheeks and forehead and these gradually increased to include her body and arms. Sarah's mother was not surprised by the eczema as she herself had ▶▶

eczema for most of her life, although it was now very mild and only affected her hands and arms. She did take Sarah to her GP who prescribed an emollient and a bath oil. Over the first few years of Sarah's life the eczema was very widespread and caused Sarah a lot of discomfort and her mother became convinced that there must be something more she could do to help find out what caused the flare-ups that occurred every so often.

Sarah's mother tried several different types of washing powder in case Sarah's eczema was related to an allergic reaction to this, but felt this made little or no difference to Sarah's eczema. Next, she tried to keep a food diary to identify whether there were any food triggers that made the eczema worse. She did not find this very helpful because the range of foods Sarah ate was quite varied and changed day-to-day, so it was impossible to identify any triggers. She then tried cleaning the house meticulously and covered Sarah's mattress and pillow with special covers to reduce her exposure to house dust mite. For a while Sarah's eczema did seem to improve; however, Sarah's mother was never convinced that this improvement was related to the cleaning, and found it very hard to keep up her enthusiasm for the work that was required. However, she did keep Sarah's bedding as free of house dust mite as possible. Following the recommendation of a friend, Sarah's mother did take her to visit a homeopath and found this consultation quite helpful. She carried out the treatment recommended, but when the tablets ran out she did not return for further treatment as Sarah's eczema had recently flared up again, and she had to treat the resulting infection using conventional antibiotics.

Sarah's mother was very reluctant to use any steroid cream on Sarah as a baby. She remembered all the warnings about the side effects of steroids that she had been given as a child. However, after a particularly bad flare she agreed to try a mild steroid and after that found it was helpful to use this occasionally. Sarah was eventually referred to a dermatology clinic and her mother found ▶

the consultation with a specialist nurse particularly helpful and she was able to improve her management of Sarah's eczema following her advice.

Gradually, over time, Sarah's eczema did reduce in severity as had her mother's. Sarah's mother found it easier to manage the eczema as Sarah grew up and was able to cooperate with treatment. She remained unclear about what caused the periodic flare-ups in Sarah's eczema, and never felt she had fully understood the causes of these.

Summary

- It can be hard to work out what is the best way of treating your child's eczema. This is partly because of the way eczema changes over time, and partly because you may be given lots of different advice.

- The conventional treatments for eczema are effective in controlling symptoms but do not necessarily lead to a cure.

- It can be difficult to stick consistently to the best possible treatment routine because it is time-consuming and has to be repeated frequently.

- There are several different types of complementary therapy which offer treatment for eczema, but it can be hard to find out how effective these are.

The impact of eczema on your child and on the family

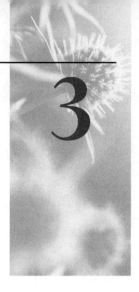

3

<blockquote>
" They aren't really that sympathetic. I think ... unless they have eczema or live with anybody with eczema, I don't think they can really understand how horrible it is. **"**
</blockquote>

<blockquote>
" Everything is forward thinking with her. Her bandages, her creams ... where to go on holiday, what you can do when you go there ... it's constant forward thinking. It does affect your whole day-to-day activities. **"**
</blockquote>

<blockquote>
" It does cause arguments with your partner too, because there is stress, terrible amounts of stress ... I think the public should be made more aware of eczema. It's a very serious disease ... it can devastate families. **"**
</blockquote>

As we have already seen, eczema is a very common condition in childhood. For many children it is also a temporary one and, even in the most severe forms of eczema, it is not life-threatening. However, eczema has a very marked effect on the quality of life of both children with eczema and their families. Why is this?

Eczema is so common it is sometimes seen as almost 'normal' or trivial. Everyone knows someone with eczema – it is not rare or exotic. However, despite this you may feel that other people don't seem to understand what it is really like for you caring for your child. This is partly because of the variation in severity of eczema. Mild eczema *is* very common and usually transient. However, chronic severe eczema is much more rare, so your friends are much less likely to come across it.

However, nearly everyone who has had the experience of caring for a child with chronic severe eczema will be very sympathetic – and will share with you that sense of eczema affecting many aspects of your life. Although many people think that the main problems with eczema are itching and scratching, the full impact of the condition is hidden. It is not a simple skin condition as it might at first appear. Eczema can affect many areas of family life: sleeping, eating, going on holiday, your child's behaviour, finances, your relationship with your partner, your household chores and even your leisure. Problems with sleeping, eating, scratching and teasing are dealt with in later chapters. This chapter covers the impact of eczema on your child and your family, your relationship with any other children you have, and with your partner.

Your relationship with your child

Eczema causes the sort of discomfort which is not easily relieved and which is chronic rather than acute: the discomfort caused by itching and the constant effort to overcome the desire to scratch is very draining over time. Babies or young children with eczema often appear slightly 'on edge' all the time. They are often very slightly irritable, except when they are distracted by interesting things happening. They often need a good deal more attention to keep them content and to help them feel comfortable.

Parents of children with eczema also often describe themselves as 'being on edge'. You may feel you are in a state of constant watchfulness – never quite able to relax and always having to think and plan ahead to manage the eczema. Rather than being able to react spontaneously you may feel you have to do everything in a planned and organised way. All sorts of environmental situations may affect your child which others would not even consider, for example a hot room, or a house with several cats in it. Even something that should be enjoyable, such as going away on holiday, can feel like a major obstacle course.

The natural history of eczema is that it is usually at its worst when your child is young, mostly in their pre-school years. As any parent of a pre-school child knows, this can be a very demanding time. As well as having to manage all the 'normal' demands of caring for a young child, you have to manage the demands of the eczema as well. Once your child does reach school age you then have to consider how to best manage his or her eczema at school, which is an added concern in addition to all the other concerns of helping a child settle into school. Although it can be hard work caring for a young child with eczema because of all these extra demands, it is important to recognise that you need to try and treat your child as you would other children of his or her age in terms of managing their behaviour, in order to minimise the impact of the eczema on their development.

My 3-year-old child has always had quite severe eczema, and I think I have always treated her more gently because I have felt so sorry for her. However, my family says that she is just spoilt and that I have made a rod for my own back. I find it hard to be firm with her when she is so unhappy and uncomfortable, but sometimes I feel so cross with her that I hate her. What should I do?

Any parent who has a child who has special needs of any form, whether this is because of a physical disability, a chronic illness or a learning disability, has a difficult juggling act on their hands in terms of how to manage their child's behaviour. On the one hand, you have to try and treat the child 'as normally as possible', but on the other hand, you do have to be sensitive to the child's additional needs as a result of his or her eczema. So how can you judge what is 'as normal as possible' for your child?

The crucial features of managing behaviour in young children are confidence in yourself as a parent and having a good, loving relationship with your child. Young children do not have the ability or the sense to know what is best for them. They think in a very short-term way and tend to respond to what feels right now. As a consequence, parents have to assume control for longer-term planning and routine. But young children can be very determined and they are not inhibited by the social embarrassment that we as adults feel. So you will often find yourself having to exert your authority over a 2- or 3-year-old who is absolutely determined to do what he or she wants and will if necessary use force or tactics such as screaming or kicking, etc., to ensure he or she gets it.

In these sorts of situations parents often lose confidence in their ability to manage their young child. (This is not helped by passers-by who feel free to comment on how badly the parent is managing!) You can also undermine your own confidence by your own thoughts about your child. If you feel guilty about upsetting your child, or if you somehow excuse the behaviour to yourself, or if you are trying to compensate because you feel sorry for your child, then you are soon going to lose confidence and 'give in'.

At this age it can often feel that you are in a 'battle of wills' with your child. But it is important to understand why your child is behaving in this way, and to accept that this is a normal process for her at this age. She is not doing these things on purpose to upset you and actually reacts in a very immediate way rather than in a planned or organised way to situations. During this difficult time remember that your child will flourish in the long term if you can help her to 'learn' the rules of social behaviour and set appropriate boundaries and routines. In the short term you might feel better by giving in to try and make your child happy, but you are not helping your child in the long run.

Even children with eczema, who might well be more tired and irritable than the average child, and for whom you may well feel sorry, have to learn these same lessons. Even parents of children with eczema, who probably do feel more exhausted and lacking in energy than parents of healthy children, have to keep up their confidence in managing their child's behaviour.

HELPFUL TIPS! HELPFUL TIPS! HELPFUL TIPS! HELPFUL

The following techniques are most helpful for young children, from about 2 years old up to 8 years old.

- Start by building up your relationship with your child so that you can begin to enjoy time with her again. You can do this by simply setting aside a small amount of time to play with her and concentrate on her. Your aim should be to get back to having fun with your child, rather than feeling you are constantly battling with her. This really does only have to be a few minutes a day to start with. Try not to be critical in this time and try not to dismiss this as irrelevant if you are battling for the other 10 hours in the day. Try to be able to forget all the other difficult things that have happened and simply try and enjoy being with your child again.

- Then begin to tackle any difficult behaviour by being firm and consistent. Decide what rules are important and enforce these consistently. Some aspects of difficult behaviour can be ignored and it is not worth fighting every single battle. For example, you can ignore cross words and most tantrums but should not ignore deliberately kicking or hitting others. Decide on your priorities and stick to these.

- When you have decided that you are going to stick to something then remember that your child will not understand that you have suddenly decided to become firm and will try her hardest to get you to give in. Because of this, it often feels that the situation gets worse before it gets better. Once your child has realised that you really do mean what you say and that you are not going to give in, then she will gradually learn it is not worth challenging you on the main rules. She may still of course ▶

continue to do other things that are difficult for you, but at least she will have stopped the worst types of behaviour.

- Make a real effort to praise your child when she does something good or something you like. It is very easy to forget that all children, even ones who have frequent tantrums, do manage to do something well every day and it is important for you to notice this and praise your child for this. Otherwise it is too easy to get caught in a negative spiral with your child, so that you spend all your time feeling cross with her, and she spends the whole day either being ignored or being told off. Noticing the positive things your child does helps to repair your relationship and helps the child to find a way out of the negative spiral.

All of these techniques are easier to do in theory than in practice. You may well need extra help to put into practice some of these ideas and to think of good ways of managing specific incidents. In particular, if you feel that you cannot use these ideas because your relationship with your child has got too difficult, or because you cannot find the energy to put them into place, then you will need extra support. There are several very good books that are easily available which give more details about how to manage difficult behaviour in this age group. (See 'Recommended further reading' at the back of the book.)

Alternatively, you can talk to your health visitor or GP about the services that are available in your area for young children with behavioural difficulties. These do vary a lot over the country so you will have to find out about your local service, but they are likely to involve health visitors, child psychologists or other professionals with expertise in working with young children. These sorts of difficulties are very common in young childhood and you should be able to get some help with managing difficult behaviour.

Your relationship with your other children

I feel that my whole life revolves around my child with eczema. I constantly feel guilty because I am not able to give the other children as much time as I would like and am often bad-tempered with them

It is always difficult in families when one member of the family needs a lot of time and attention and the other members feel like they are missing out. It is not always possible to 'share yourself out' evenly, but it feels unfair if you have to focus on one child or you find you take short cuts with the others simply because you feel exhausted and have run out of energy. Some children pick up on this and it is particularly difficult if you feel your child is then using this as ammunition in other battles. You may find your other children seem to be vying for your attention in other ways, by being uncharacteristically demanding or taking advantage of your lack of time.

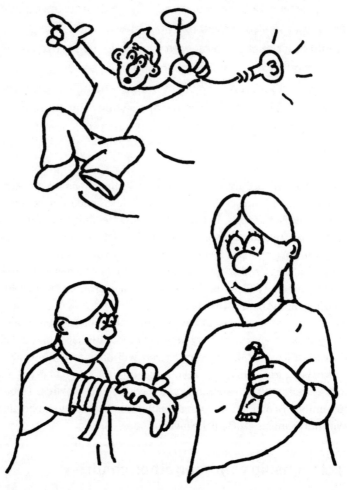

It can be hard to find time for your other children.

Although it is hard, you have to accept that caring for a child with chronic eczema is a time-consuming business and it may not be the case that you are failing to use your time efficiently, but that you do have only just enough time and energy to cope. Try very hard to think of any short cuts you can use to help you devote more time to the things that you consider your priority rather than having your time absorbed by trivial or repetitive tasks that anyone else can do. It is not necessarily easy to find a substitute for you in terms of childcare, but there are ways of other people substituting for you for other tasks such as cleaning, shopping, etc. It can be hard to accept offers of help from others and you may feel that you should be able to manage on your own. But if you do get offers of help, don't feel that you have to manage on your own.

Very few parents feel they are able to do the best for all of their children all the time. Everyone has limitations and there are times when other factors make it impossible to spend as much time as you would want to with your children. Rather than feeling guilty and critical of what you do manage, it is helpful to make a conscious effort to do one small thing with each of your other children every day. During this time you have to make this your child's special time. Focus on your child and don't be 'mentally' absent, for example thinking through all the chores you will have to do later. This really only needs to be for about 5 or 10 minutes, but make it a special time for your child. Make sure you use it on an activity that will give you some good quality time with your child – not just an additional time to nag at them to tidy away their toys.

When most parents start doing this they think that they already spend this sort of time with their child but what is different is that this is time to focus on the needs of your child rather than fitting them in among all the other demands you have on your time. Having then spent just a few minutes of every day you will be giving each child a small amount of you which will help preserve your relationship with them, while you go through the difficult time of sharing out your time between everyone and everything else.

Your relationship with your partner

I feel like I'm the only one in our family who really takes responsibility for my child's eczema. I wish my partner would understand what a difficult time it is for me and be less demanding himself

When you have been caring for a young child it can feel hard to respond positively to your partner at the end of the day. This can easily lead to difficulties between couples because of the lack of good time for each other and the potential resentment that can build up on either side.

It has traditionally been the mother who has been the main carer for children in the family. This is gradually changing over time, but it is still the case that for the vast majority of families it is the mother who carries the responsibility for caring for the children when they are unwell or have a chronic illness. For some families, this is fine and seen as an acceptable division of labour. However, for others, particularly when the partners have been very equal before having children, it can feel 'unfair' when one is left with this responsibility. When there is a child with a chronic illness in the family, the more traditional roles often predominate.

There are times in family life, particularly when children are very young, when it feels that there simply isn't enough time in the day and some things have to go. Gradually as the children get older, it becomes possible to go back to old interests or to start new ones, but for a while it feels like there is no space and time for each parent as an individual, let alone as a couple. This is exacerbated when the partners are tired or stressed or simply going through a very busy time. It is a difficult time for many couples and it requires give and take on both sides. It is too easy to let resentments build up and to avoid the real underlying problems. If you feel you need help you should be able to ask for it. It can become even harder, however, when you both have completely different expectations of each other and aren't able to negotiate this.

Some children can also be very controlling of who they will accept doing their treatment. For example, if their mother becomes more and more skilled at doing the treatment and this routine becomes more and more familiar, the child might be reluctant to accept another carer stepping in to help. This can undermine the confidence of the partner and make it tempting for him to hand back care to the mother. It can also be very tempting for the mother to become unwilling to try and let her partner help out because it feel easier to 'just do it' or because there is a part of her is pleased that she has become the 'expert' at this. Some mothers also get a sense of pride from their mastery of the child's treatment and may be reluctant to let go of this. This pattern often develops over time: the family start out with good intentions of sharing some of the care, but as time goes by, sharing happens less and less and eventually it ends up with the mother doing all the care.

Remember that the rules of who should do what are not written in stone. Check out with each other about what you do consider acceptable and be honest when you feel angry or resentful about what your partner is doing or not doing. These difficulties are hard to overcome because it is likely that both of you are under different stresses, but if resentment is allowed to build up it will just become increasingly difficult to tackle.

Problem behaviour

My child can't sit still and concentrate for more than a minute. Is my child hyperactive?

Attention Deficit Hyperactivity Disorder (ADHD) is the term given to a form of behavioural difficulties in children. Children with ADHD are extremely physically active, for example constantly fidgeting, constantly in and out of their seat at the table during meals, unable to sit still in a classroom situation. In addition, they find it hard to concentrate on tasks and hard to complete work that has been set. They may start work but then forget what they are supposed to be doing and get very easily distracted by things around them. Children with ADHD also find it hard to control their impulses and may therefore do quite dangerous things without appearing to understand that they are putting themselves at risk. ADHD is more common among boys than girls and affects up to 3 per cent of children.

The reason the diagnosis of ADHD is controversial is because, as you can see from the description, it all depends how severe it is. Many children, particularly boys, *are* quite physically restless and active when they are young and they do find it hard to settle in a classroom situation at the age of five. However, it is only when these problems are quite severe that the child has true ADHD. In addition there has been a lot of publicity about the use of medication to control the symptoms of children with ADHD. This is quite a new treatment and, whereas there were virtually no children receiving this sort of treatment 10 years ago, it is becoming more and more widely used. However, the medication that is used, methylphenidate (often known under the brand name of Ritalin), like all other types of medication, has side effects and is not a perfect cure for all the problems associated with ADHD. It does help to control the symptoms for some children, but it has to be used properly and supervised by an appropriately qualified and experienced children's doctor, usually a community paediatrician or a child psychiatrist. It is important to be realistic about the use of this sort of medication before embarking on assessment for ADHD, because too many parents hope that if a diagnosis is made, the child's problems will be solved. Unfortunately, the medication does not work in that way and should be thought of as a useful way of controlling symptoms for some children with extremely marked hyperactivity in the particular situations in which their concentration and attention difficulties cause problems, which is nearly always at school.

Some studies have suggested that children with eczema have high rates of ADHD. However, it appears that this is at least partly because of the overlap between the symptoms of ADHD and the restlessness often seen in children with eczema because of the discomfort they experience. Some children with eczema are very fidgety and restless, they do find it hard to concentrate and they do get easily distracted. However, this is usually caused by their skin condition rather than underlying hyperactivity. Of course, there will be some children with ADHD who also have eczema, so it is important to consider both how the eczema affects the child and how severe the symptoms are in terms of deciding whether a child has ADHD.

If you are concerned about your child's ability to concentrate and to focus on tasks, you can ask your GP to refer to your local child development service or your local child mental health service for an assessment. Also, you can ask your child's teacher about your concerns because they usually have a good idea of what is in the 'normal' range for your child's age group, and if they feel your child is outside the 'normal' range then that is a helpful bit of information for your local service. As part of the assessment process it will probably be necessary to assess your child both on a one-to-one basis and in a group situation, usually at school. You may well be offered advice about how to manage your child's behaviour without using medication, using behavioural techniques. Although these are hard work, they are important because, even if you child does have ADHD, you will be able to learn more effective ways of managing difficult behaviour at home.

My child is very shy. How can I help him become more outgoing and confident?

Just as with levels of hyperactivity, children vary in how socially confident they feel and how shy they are with other people. On average, research studies have shown that children with eczema are more likely to be at the quiet and shy end of the spectrum than at the extrovert end of the spectrum. This is also true for children with other types of physical health problems.

Most children who are shy do not need any attention drawn to this. Putting them on the spot or criticising them for being shy can make them feel even more self-conscious and less confident. Saying to a child who is shy, 'Has the cat got your tongue?', does not usually help them to feel more comfortable to speak out. Most children who are shy do gradually become more confident once they have had the chance to get to know the children and adults around them. So it is important to help them to build up confidence in difficult situations rather than expecting them to speak out when they do not feel confident in themselves. After all, group situations would be impossible to manage if absolutely every child was outgoing and extrovert. Groups work best when there is a combination of different personalities, some quiet and reserved children as well as the bouncy, outgoing ones.

It is important to ensure that your child does have the skills necessary to manage the things he or she is expected to do as part of normal development (such as beginning to manage away from his or her main carer at nursery or playgroup). It is also important not to let other people treat them as a doormat. Acknowledging that they are shy helps, but then they need help with very specific skills in situations in which they need to be able to present themselves. For example, if they are going to have to say a few lines in the school play, they may need extra help practising this.

Shyness is really only a problem when it prevents a child from making the most of their potential. A shy child will never become a confident actor, but that is not likely to be a problem because few shy children want to become actors.

However they will have to be able to manage some social situations and so they may need help to develop specific skills for situations such as presenting a piece of work in school.

If you feel your child's shyness is closely linked to embarrassment about their physical appearance because of their eczema, then it is important for them to develop their self-esteem. Contrary to popular belief, physical appearance is not the most important determinant of happiness. There are many people who are very popular and happy, although they are not physically the best-looking, because of their personality. It may be hard to convince your child of this because of the way we are inundated with images of beauty and because of the way beauty is so highly valued in the media. Nonetheless self-esteem is more than just feeling good about the way you look, and you can encourage your child to feel good about him or herself in many ways. This is covered in more detail in Chapter 7.

The financial impact of eczema

Having a child with eczema can place an additional financial burden on the family. One recent study suggested that childhood eczema may cost as much as £47 m a year in the UK and that the cost to the family is about a third of this total. Some of these additional costs are directly attributable to the eczema; for example, you may end up buying some types of cream yourself, or you may have the additional expense of buying treatments that are not routinely available through the NHS, for example homeopathic remedies. Other expenses include buying suitable clothing that might be more expensive than you would normally buy, such as cotton clothes, or replacing clothes frequently because of the way the creams destroy clothes. Less obviously, you may incur extra costs because you are unable to work as you would with a healthy child, or because you have to replace your washing machine more frequently because the oils and creams rot the rubber seals and tubes.

In some situations it is possible to claim Disability Living Allowance which is a type of benefit that does not depend on your income. The basis of your claim would be the level of additional care your child needs as a consequence of his or her eczema. This benefit reflects the additional care burden of caring for a child with some form of illness or disability and therefore requires a considerable amount of detailed information about the sort of care your child requires. If you want to find our more about this benefit you can get further information from the Benefits Agency (see 'Useful addresses and contacts' at the back of the book). The forms are quite long and daunting, but you can get help filling out the forms from the Benefits Agency or from a hospital social worker (if your child is receiving hospital care).

CASE STUDY CASE STUDY CASE STUDY CASE STUDY

Connor

Connor was a healthy baby but developed eczema when he was about 4 months old. He had a sister who was 2 years older than him who did not have any health problems. When Connor was nearly 2, his behaviour became harder and harder to manage. He had always been a physically active baby and as soon as he was able to move around, he would be constantly 'on the go' and climbing on and off things around the house. He had frequent temper tantrums whenever his mother tried to stop him doing things and his mother found his behaviour very hard to manage.

Connor's eczema was mostly on his arms and legs by this time and, although it was quite well controlled, he often appeared uncomfortable and would sit scratching himself while playing. He also appeared very restless and would rarely settle to play with one toy for more than a few minutes at a time before moving on to the next.

Connor's parents and grandparents often commented on how different he was to his sister who had been a much more settled and contented child and had shown good concentration. She was now at nursery and enjoyed being with other children and could sit and listen to stories or settle to do colouring or painting. Connor on the other hand found it difficult to share with other children and when other children came to play he would often end up over-excited and become very disobedient.

At the time, Connor's mother found managing his behaviour a constant strain and did not enjoy spending time with him. His father could enjoy playing with Connor for a short while, but this often ended with either his father getting angry or Connor getting over-excited. Over the next 2 years Connor's eczema gradually improved. However, his behaviour remained very difficult to

▶

manage. His mother attended a parenting course run by a local health visitor and found some of the suggestions very helpful. In particular she realised that she had rather unrealistic expectations for Connor because his sister had been so easy to manage and had rarely challenged her. She became more consistent with him, for example, ensuring that when she said 'no' she didn't then give in 5 minutes later. She also changed the way she structured her time to fit in with his ability to concentrate. She no longer expected him to occupy himself for more than a few minutes at a time, and tried to plan ahead rather than just responding when things went wrong.

Gradually, Connor's ability to concentrate began to improve with age. His mother began to feel more positively towards him and found that she could enjoy doing things with him. Although he was still a very physically active boy who easily became over-excited, he began to make some friendships and to learn how to cooperate with other children.

Summary

- Eczema can have a marked impact on many aspects of family life.

- It can be difficult to juggle the needs of your child with eczema with the needs of the other members of the family.

- Maintain your relationship with all your children by playing with them or doing some short activity with them.

- Use lots of praise and notice when things go well.

- Be firm and consistent about your rules.

- Keep negotiating with your partner – don't let resentments build up.

Understanding and managing scratching

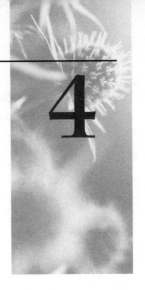

4

"I can't bear it when she scratches, I can't bear it."

"The last three nights she has got so tired that she has started to give cheek and really misbehave and then she actually said to me last night, 'Right, that's it then, I'm just going to scratch,' and that's only because we had an argument about something else. But it was like a weapon then. So I just said, 'Right, there's nothing I can do about that, I'm going downstairs.'"

"He seems like he's almost in a daze. You can't get him to stop, you can't reason with him. If I try and hold him to stop him he will get frantic. It scares me seeing him like that."

Why do children scratch?

Scratching is the natural response to the sensation of itching that your child feels as a consequence of eczema. However, although scratching is the natural response to itching, scratching actually damages the skin and makes the itch worse. A vicious circle develops – itching leads to scratching which leads to skin damage which leads to more itching and then to more scratching. This is often called the 'itch–scratch cycle'.

For most children the immediate sense of relief they get from scratching far outweighs any attempt to persuade them not to scratch. Children think in the here and now and in the short term. If it feels good and takes away the unpleasant feeling of the itch they will scratch. It is extremely hard to persuade a young child who is feeling itchy that scratching will only make things worse in the long term – they know that in the short term it does feel better. Even adults find this hard and frequently succumb to the temptation of having a scratch, knowing that this will be harmful in the long run.

'Scratching' can take many forms. Rather than scratching with their fingers, babies and young children often rub the itchy part of their body. They are sometimes unaware they are doing this and the determination shown by a young baby when he or she is trying to rub itchy skin can be phenomenal. Older children learn other ways of scratching, such as using an object to rub against themselves – for example a ruler or a comb. They will use the edges of furniture or any other convenient object to scratch against.

How can I help my child not to scratch?

The most effective way of reducing scratching is to reduce the amount of itching your child feels. Make sure your treatment regime is as good as it can possibly be. Make sure you have controlled as many of the factors that lead to itching as possible. Controlling the causes of itching will make a big difference to the amount of scratching your child does.

Teach your child alternatives to scratching as soon as possible. Obviously babies and young children do not have the capacity to use these sorts of techniques, but as your child gets older encourage them to try alternatives. Rather then scratching, they can use one finger to press on the itchy part. This is much less damaging than scratching and does give some relief from the itchy feeling. Or they can gently pinch the skin for a few moments.

As your child gets older you can then teach them even better substitute activities that keep their hands occupied without damaging their skin at all. For example, when they feel the need to scratch they can try doing alternative things with their hands until the itchy sensation decreases. They can squeeze their hand into a tightly clenched fist and hold that for a count of 30. They can carry around 'worry beads' in their pocket and use these to keep their hands occupied for a few minutes. Try to encourage them to 'keep their hands occupied' whenever they feel itchy.

Why shouldn't I say, 'Don't scratch!'?

You will often be advised never to say, 'Don't scratch!' This is partly because it is unlikely your child will take much notice if they are already scratching and partly because, if they do stop temporarily, they will probably try again later – probably hidden away from you so that you can't see them.

But, most importantly, it is also because most children (and adults) do not respond well to being told to stop doing something. It is often much easier to persuade them to *do* something else than to *stop* doing something. Children with chronic eczema experience many, many episodes of being told not to scratch. Just like any other form of nagging, it really does stop registering with your child after a while, except as another form of annoyance.

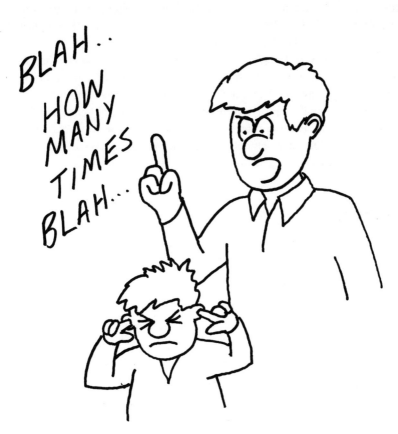

Saying 'don't scratch' can be counterproductive.

However, there must be very few parents of children with chronic eczema who can honestly say they have been able to stick to this advice all the time. Even with the best of intentions, there will be times when your patience snaps and you blurt out something along the lines of 'Stop scratching!' If you find you are doing this a lot, or are feeling like you are losing control, you need to start again and find a better way of managing your own reaction to scratching.

My child gets furious with me if I try and stop her scratching. She seems to get enormous pleasure out of the sensation of scratching. What can I do?

It can be extremely distressing to see a child in a 'scratching frenzy'. They become absorbed in the sensation caused by scratching and sometimes appear as though they are in a trance. Some parents describe this as almost like some type of drug – the child is totally caught up in the physical sensation. By the time you get your child out of the frenzy they may have done a lot of damage to their skin including breaking their skin so it is bleeding.

They best way of dealing with scratching frenzies is to do as much as you can to prevent them. Prevention is better than cure but it is also a lot of hard work, which is why we all find it so hard to do in practice. But once a child is in a frenzy, they will not listen to reason and they will not find it easy to stop. It really is worth investing extra time and energy to prevent these as much as possible because the damage done in a frenzy can take days to heal. Develop an action plan for dealing with scratching bouts and put it into practice with determination.

HELPFUL TIPS! HELPFUL TIPS! HELPFUL TIPS! HELPFUL

If your child is about 3 years old or older, you can begin to involve them in this:

- In a calm moment, not when the child is scratching, let your child know your plan of action for dealing with these bouts of scratching. Tell them firmly and in a caring way that you are going to help them when they feel like this. Talk to them about your strategy and make it very concrete and specific. It helps to break it down into steps. For example, step one may be to simply say to them, 'I can see you are getting itchy. Let's get your (favourite toy)'. At this point you have a chance of distracting them, so put a lot of energy into this. Although it feels like huge effort, its probably going to pay off later.

- If your first attempt at distracting doesn't seem to have much effect, you have to move on to more active ways of distracting your child. Step two might be taking the child out of the situation and doing something jointly with him for 10 minutes. You will ▶

have to work hard to find something that is interesting enough to distract your child, and it will therefore require a lot of energy and effort on your part.

- If this is still not enough then step three might be putting your child into the bath and actively playing with him to both distract him and help treat the itching.

- If despite all your efforts, your child ends up in a scratching frenzy, keep calm and do not let yourself get in a frenzy too. You may need to use some calming techniques yourself to help yourself do this. As soon as you see any signs of your child calming go and cuddle him and gently hold him as he calms down. Do not shout and do not start saying, 'Look what you've done to your skin!' however tempting it might be. Many children do feel quite upset when they realise how much they have hurt themselves and you should help your child understand that this is a problem for him or her as well as you. Use this opportunity to talk about trying to help prevent this happening again.

How can I keep calm?

There are several times in this book when it is suggested that it is important to 'keep calm'. Whilst this may be the best way of managing many childhood problems (for example, difficult behaviour, sleep problems, scratching, etc.) it is extremely hard to do. Often when we lose our composure it is not the event itself that has triggered the outburst, it is the build-up of tension beforehand, and the actual event itself may be quite minor. Many parents admit that the times that they smack their child it is not because of what the child has done on that particular occasion, it is a build-up of tension beforehand. The child's behaviour is simply 'the straw that breaks the camel's back'.

If you are finding it extremely difficult to keep calm then it might be worth trying to think through what is going on in the background that has led to the build-up of tension. For example, did you get furious with your child when he was scratching in the back of the car more because you were annoyed with the traffic, than with the scratching? Did you shout at your child in the night when he woke you up because you felt it wasn't your turn to get up again and your partner was fast asleep?

HELPFUL TIPS! HELPFUL TIPS! HELPFUL TIPS! HELPFUL

- If you are finding it hard to keep calm, try and take stock of what is happening and why it is hard to keep calm.

- Remember that we have the responsibility as the adult in the situation not to take it out on our children. We cannot expect our children to act reasonably and respond to rules consistently if we react in illogical and frightening ways towards them.

- Take a deep breath, concentrate on breathing out and relaxing your shoulders. Do this three times.

- If the situation is safe, walk away rather than overreact. This is especially important if you think you might hit your child out of anger. It is often better simply to leave your child on his or her own for a few minutes than to overreact.

I sometimes think that my child scratches automatically and that is has become a habit for her. How can I change this?

All scratching does start off as a response to itching. However, over time, scratching can take on a life of its own and become more of a habit, like thumb-sucking or nail-biting. The scratching itself may well then become a very important factor in maintaining the eczema, and the scratching can even become the major cause of the skin damage, rather than the eczema itself.

We all know how common habits are, and how hard they are to break. However, there are some well-established techniques that have been shown to be very effective in breaking habits and these can be used with scratching too. These techniques are known as 'habit reversal' and although they are most effective with adults, they can be used with some modification with children as well. The difficulty with applying them to children is that the child herself has to want to change the behaviour, not just her parent. If your child does not see the logic in trying to reduce scratching, or is not at all motivated to try and reduce it, these techniques will not work.

There are ways of increasing your child's motivation which are used for bringing about any form of behaviour change in a child (such as sitting at the table for meals, or brushing their teeth every day, or reducing temper outbursts). These take the form of rewards. Young children, particularly under 4 years old, need very immediate rewards and so it is quite hard to use these techniques with them. However, children aged four to nine often respond very well to reward charts, often known as 'star charts'. The child is given a sticker for successfully completing whatever the behaviour we want from them, and can earn a bigger reward for successfully collecting a certain number of stars. You can use some sort of reward chart to help your child become more motivated to use the habit reversal techniques.

Star charts have to be used properly to be successful in changing behaviour and there are certain ways of making a star chart more effective. Firstly, involve your child in making the actual chart, choosing the stickers and deciding on the rewards. We want them to be interested in it! Secondly, carefully choose the behaviour for which they will be rewarded. Don't put it negatively (for example, don't choose 'not scratching') but put it as a positive behaviour ('pinching the itch'). Carefully choose the time over which the behaviour is expected to happen. If you say, you must 'pinch the itch' for the whole day he or she is unlikely to succeed. Instead, break the day down into sections. For example, one star for the time before school, another star for when they get home to when they finish tea, and another for the evening including bathtime. It is essential the child gets some reward early on otherwise they will lose interest. Star charts do not work forever, so put a lot of effort into making it work for about two or three weeks. It is also essential to choose rewards that your child is highly motivated to achieve. These do not have to be things that cost a lot (although many children are motivated by these). They can be extra privileges, such as being allowed to stay up and watch a special TV programme with both parents. Or they can be like a 'dare', for example agreeing to allow them to dye their hair a particular colour (temporarily).

If your use a reward chart together with a habit reversal programme, you may find you can motivate your child enough to learn some useful techniques for reducing scratching.

Habit reversal programme

The first step in changing a habit is to become aware of the behaviour again. Once a behaviour has become a habit it is done unconsciously without the person even being aware they are doing it. So the first step in changing the habit is simply to record every time it happens. You can do this in various different ways. If your child is quite young, you can keep a diary for a few days while you observe him or her. Just keep a count or a tally of scratching episodes and note down any situations that might be relevant. In the example in Box 2, each tally indicates one period of five minutes that included scratching.

Box 2.	Example of a scratching diary.
7:00	
7:30	Scratching while watching cartoons on TV |||
8:00	Breakfast
8:30	Scratching while changing into uniform ||
9:00	School
3:30	Pick him up
4:00	
4:30	Scratching while doing homework ||||
5:00	Tea
5:30	Scratching while watching TV ||
6:00	Scratching while watching TV |||
6:30	
7:00	Bath: Scratching afterwards ||

If your child is older, say eight or above, you could get her to keep a tally herself using a 'tally counter'. This is a little hand-held counter which has a button on the top and each time the button is pressed the counter increases by one. These are used in habit reversal programmes for adults and can be bought via mail order (see 'Useful addresses and contacts' at the back of the book). Each time she scratches she has to add one to the tally. This is ideal because the child herself has to recognise when the scratching occurs and begins to take some responsibility for controlling it again.

Once you have been monitoring the scratching for a week, you may well find it has started to reduce already. Simply by having to monitor habits, they do begin to reduce because we have become aware of them again. You may also find that the scratching tends to be worse at particular times of the day. This might be when the child is unoccupied, for example when watching television, or when they are feeling tired, for example at the end of the day. It is also likely to be at times when their skin is most exposed, for example when getting dressed or undressed. This will all help to plan how to reduce the scratching.

The next stage is to substitute an alternative for the scratching. The most useful techniques seem to be to those that keep the child's hands occupied and that are a close alternative to scratching, such as pinching the skin or pressing one finger hard into the itchy bit of the skin. You may need to link this new behaviour into some sort of a reward chart, as described above, in order to help your child feel more motivated to change his or her behaviour. For example, your child could earn one sticker for using the new method in the time he or she is watching TV. If your child is keen to stop scratching anyway, you might not need to introduce this extra motivation; but, if he or she does not appear very enthusiastic, then this can help to provide an incentive for doing the new behaviour.

With young children it is essential that you spend time with your child helping them to use this substitute behaviour. You also have to work hard at providing alternatives and helping to distract your child at times they find particularly difficult. This means spending more time directly with him or her than you would normally do and can be very hard to put into practice. Over time, the 'new' behaviour should happen more and more and the old habit of scratching should reduce.

Habit reversal techniques can be extremely useful in reducing habitual scratching. They do require considerable effort and motivation and the most common reason for them not working is lack of motivation. They are most effective when combined with a good skin care programme, and these two should be used hand in hand.

Box 3. Summary of habit reversal techniques.

- Record scratching: increase your child's awareness of when he or she scratches. ▶

- Design a reward system for introducing the alternative to scratching.

- Teach your child a substitute for scratching.

- Help him or her learn how to put this into practice.

- Reward your child when he or she uses the new technique.

I'm sure my child 'uses' scratching to annoy me – she knows I can't leave her to scratch and I feel manipulated by her. What can I do to change this?

Some children pick up very early on that scratching is a very effective way of getting attention and a powerful threat to use to get what they want. (This is not unique to children with eczema – children with no eczema do find other useful alternatives, such as holding their breath until they literally go blue, or refusing to eat.)

It is important to realise that the reason children do this is because it works – not because they are deliberately enjoying being manipulative or because they are a particularly nasty child, but just because it has proved to be successful. Some children fortunately never seem to make this connection and hence it doesn't occur to them to 'use' scratching in this way. Other children are very quick to pick up on the power of scratching. Just like with tantrums, there are some children who go through the whole of their pre-school years with fewer than a dozen tantrums. There are other children who will regularly have several tantrums a day. If you have the former type of child, count yourself lucky. If you have the latter type, you will need considerable determination to prevent your child using scratching as a weapon.

It is hard for any parent not to feel cross with their child when they feel 'manipulated' in this way. It is amazing how powerful and determined young children can be, and how incompetent they can make their parents feel. All parents feel judged to some extent by other people and young children can choose the moment to act up for maximum embarrassment and effectiveness. But keeping calm and not getting agitated by this sort of behaviour is very important, although admittedly hard to do.

There are ways that you can behave to make it less likely that your child is able to use scratching as an effective weapon. If you live your whole life around trying to avoid scratching and jump to attention the minute scratching starts, your child is more likely to make the connection. If you find scratching particularly upsetting and get very emotional about your child's scratching, they will find it easier to 'wind you up' and get a response by scratching than any other way.

Of course, these are not easy things to change. Most families do find that large chunks of their life are organised by a child with severe, chronic eczema. If you get very worn down and tired, you can often feel very emotional too. The key to managing this is to behave confidently and consistently and be proactive. Young children thrive on love and affection, and on knowing what the limits are. Although children will push and push to test the limits set for them, you are not doing them any favours if you are unable to stick to the limits you have set. You can see this in any well-run nursery for 2- or 3- year-olds. Very clear rules are made, and stuck to by everyone. There are clear sanctions for unacceptable behaviour, and these are used in the same way by all the members of staff.

Rather than starting with the difficult or problem behaviour, it is more important to first ensure that you improve your relationship with your child. Make sure that despite all the other demands on your time, you have some time each day when you give them your undivided attention and build up to a time when you can enjoy being together, if only for a few minutes at a time. Set aside a short time, say 10 minutes, when you can concentrate on having a good time with her. Let her choose the activity and really concentrate on making a good time for her. Try and forget about all the other things you should be (or would rather be) getting on with and focus on your child. The reason this is important is that having some good time with your child is essential when she is feeling in need of attention. Although most parents think they already do spend enough time with their child, it is not always time focused on the child and is more likely to be while you are half doing something else or not fully listening to what your child is saying.

Then act proactively if and when your child seems to be about to threaten to start scratching. Keep calm and don't show your child if you are angry or upset. Take control of the situation by redirecting your child to do something different, whilst at the same time saying to her that you won't change your mind just because she is scratching. This can be tricky if you are in a public situation and you may feel that you cannot deal with the problem then and there and have to get out of the situation first. However, if your child is able to see that she no longer gets such a response from you, then scratching will not seem quite such a powerful tool.

If you still find it very upsetting to see or hear your child scratch, particularly if it makes you feel very emotional, it is worth talking about these feelings to someone who does understand. The National Eczema Society have a helpline which is very useful if you are feeling you need more advice. Or you may feel that it would be helpful to talk to another parent who has had a similar experience. If you feel you need more than this, then talk to your GP who may be able to refer you to a counsellor or psychologist who can give you some time to talk about your own feelings and to help you think about why it is upsetting you. It is often hard to give yourself the time you need to think about how your child's eczema affects you, particularly when you are busy with young children; but it may in the long term help you to manage your child's care more effectively.

I've heard that hypnosis can help decrease scratching. How does this work?

When most of us think of hypnosis we think of the stage or television form of hypnosis that is really used as a form or entertainment. However, hypnosis can be used as a form of very deep relaxation, almost like meditation, to help reduce uncomfortable physical symptoms. It is also sometimes called 'guided imagery' because imagery is used to help change the uncomfortable physical symptoms. Many children enjoy using their imagination in this way and can get very involved with imaginary scenes or stories, so they sometimes find these sorts of techniques more accessible than adults do. Children from the age of about eight and up are best able to use these sorts of techniques as very young children do not have the concentration span necessary to make full use of the technique.

One research study was conducted at Great Ormond Street using guided imagery to help children control symptoms of itching due to eczema. There did appear to be some benefits from this type of approach, although further research does need to be done in this area.

The aim of the imagery is to help the child to reduce any sensation of itching and to replace this with a positive relaxed feeling. The process starts by developing a story, as agreed with the child in advance, to suit their own interests and preferences. A typical storyline might include a child going through a closed doorway into a beautiful secret garden in which they find a fountain. The smells, sights and feeling of being in the garden would all be described to the child to help make the image very vivid and 'alive' in the child's imagination. The child might then dip their hands into the water of the fountain and find the sprinkling of the water very soothing. The suggestion would be made that as the water is sprinkled onto the child's skin, the child feels a cool, soothing sensation and that this gradually spreads over the child's body. Standard relaxation techniques would be included in the description such as the suggestion that as you get more relaxed, you notice your breathing getting slower and slower, and that as you relax, your body feels heavier and heavier. These all help the child feel more relaxed and physically comfortable.

Other possible storylines could include going on a walk through a wood and finding a clearing in the middle of the wood with the sunlight coming in through the leaves and falling on a pond with special water in it. Or travelling on a boat across a river to a mysterious island where there is a special type of snow on the hills, and the child picks up a handful of snow and a cool and soothing feeling spreads across his or her skin.

Most children find these sorts of techniques quite strange at first; but some children very quickly get engrossed in the story and become very relaxed as a result. The ideal way to do this is to be able to discuss the sort of storyline the child would like in advance and then to do a relaxation sequence with the child, holding a hand-held tape recorder so that the sequence is recorded on a tape for the child to use again. After practising the technique several times, some children are able to use the relaxation in other contexts, such as when going to sleep. In fact, these sorts of techniques are ideally suited to helping an itchy child find a way to settle at night.

The difficulty with doing this sort of sequence yourself is that your child may find it harder to really get engaged in the process with a family member. If your child does not fully engage, or does not want to try these sorts of techniques, it is hard for you to persuade them. These techniques do require a bit of mental effort, so do not suit all children.

It is worth noting that some parents of children with eczema also enjoy these types of relaxation sequences and find the techniques very useful, for example in the middle of the night, when you have just had to sort out your itchy child and are trying to get back to sleep yourself. In particular the use of breathing exercises to focus on breathing out and using the suggestion of getting more and more relaxed with each breath out can be a short cut to calm down in a tense or difficult situation.

Box 4. **Example of a script for a relaxation sequence and guided imagery.**

Start by getting yourself into a comfortable position and close your eyes so you can really concentrate on what I am saying. We're going to start by going through all your muscle groups and gradually relaxing each set of muscles. Let's start with your hands. Close your hand up tightly into a fist and hold it really tight for a few moments. Pull your fingers in really tight and make your hand into a hard fist. Now, let go, let your fingers flop open and completely relax your whole hand. Notice how different it feels from when it was tightly closed. Let your hands rest down and feel how heavy they are now.

Now let's move on to your arms. Tighten up all your arm muscles and make your arms go really hard and tight. Hold them tightly for a few ▶

moments and then let your arms go, relaxing down by your sides. As you relax, breathe out slowly and let your body begin to sink downwards as you breathe out.

(Repeat this for other areas of the body: shoulders, tummy and bottom, legs and feet.)

Now notice how much more relaxed your whole body has become and how heavy you now feel. Each time you breathe out, let yourself sink down into your chair and get comfortable so we can concentrate on your special place.

Imagine you can see in front of you a large wooden door with a big handle. Turn the handle and open the door and step through to the other side. As you step through the door you feel gentle, warm air on your face and you can see in front of you a beautiful garden. The garden is full of beautiful plants and you can see flowers of lots of different colours. Underneath your feet you can feel the soft green grass and the ground feels firm but soft under your feet. As you look around the garden you notice that there are lots of flowers of different colours as well as the green of the grass and the bushes. A short distance in front of you, you can see a water fountain and can hear the sound of the water gently splashing as it falls downwards from the fountain. You walk forwards to the fountain and dip your hands into the water which is just at a perfect temperature. The water feels refreshing and comfortable on your skin and you feel very comfortable and calm as you stand there with your hands in the water. Notice how that sense of comfort spreads all over your body and you feel happy and relaxed standing there. Remember that feeling you have now, because whenever you want to get back to feeling this comfortable again all you have to do is to remember this garden and how you have felt here today. Just enjoy being here and take a moment to remember all the things you can see, hear and feel in the garden. Remember that this is your special garden and that you can come back here yourself whenever you want.

(Add to this detail as necessary.)

Now we're going to have to leave the garden so I want you to turn around away from the fountain and to begin to walk back to the door we came through. Remember you can come back when you want but for now we are leaving the garden. Try and stay as relaxed as you are now as you go back up to the door. Reach out for the handle and open the door so that you can walk back through to the other side.

▶

Now gradually bring your mind back to the room we are in and try and keep as comfortable and relaxed as you are now. When you are ready, open your eyes again and bring your mind back into this room. Just allow yourself a few moments to adjust to being in the room again.

Summary

- Scratching can lead to skin damage and results in the 'itch–scratch cycle'.

- It is important not to overreact to scratching, even if it upsets you.

- Work hard to prevent your child getting into a scratching frenzy.

- If scratching has become a 'habit', try using habit reversal techniques to teach your child an alternative to scratching.

- Use guided imagery to help your child learn physical relaxation techniques.

Understanding and managing sleep problems

5

> **"**I just long for a night of uninterrupted sleep – I feel like I'm a robot. I can only just keep going and have no energy for trying anything new.**"**

> **"**I hate it when she wakes up and I have to try and keep myself calm and try to help her to calm down. Sometimes I think I can't bear it, I can't do it, but I do because I have no choice. Who else is going to do it?**"**

In a recent survey of members of the National Eczema Society, 60 per cent of parents of children with eczema said that the child's eczema affected their child's sleep. As well as having an impact on the child, this will inevitably also affect parents and siblings. Experiencing repeated nights of disturbed sleep is often described as a form of torture and for many families the sleep difficulties caused by eczema have a very big impact on their quality of life.

It is important to understand that sleeping problems in young children are extremely common even in healthy children. At least 25 per cent (or one in four) of 1-year-old children regularly wake at night or have difficulties settling. Although this number does decrease as children get older, at 4 years old, 10 per cent (or one in ten) still have sleep problems.

Families vary widely in their attitudes towards establishing sleep routines for their children. The most common pattern is to have a bedtime routine, which usually involves bathtime, quiet play or reading and then settling to sleep. However, some families find that this routine breaks down when they have a child with a sleep problem. If the child is hard to settle, he or she may end up spending more time up with his or her parents or bedtime gets later and later until it ends up being the same as the parents. Some families have young children sleeping in with one or both parents, either because that is what they prefer or because they feel they have no choice.

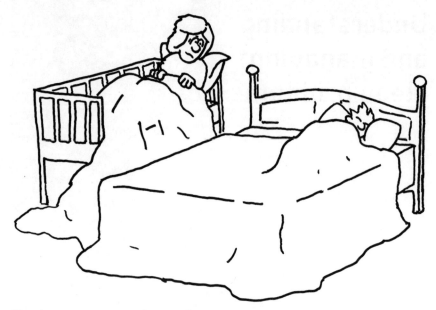

Sleeping arrangements often get disrupted when you have a child with eczema.

From the moment they are born, babies vary in their temperament. Some babies cry very little, are easy to soothe and settle and generally appear content. Other babies appear much more unsettled. They cry more and are difficult to soothe and settle. However, whatever the type of baby you have got, they are also going to be influenced from the very beginning by how they are handled and how you manage their unsettled times. As we know from the way the advice about how to manage crying has changed over time, there are 'fashions' in how to manage a baby for the best. For example, many women who are grandmothers or great-grandmothers now may well have been told that crying is an important way for the child's lungs to develop, and that they should leave their baby to cry him or herself to sleep. Mothers who had their children in the 1980s or 1990s are more likely to have been told that, because crying is the only way that a baby can communicate, you should respond straight away when they cry, and that it is impossible to spoil a baby – they need you immediately. Now there is a shift back to the importance of routines, but hopefully with more understanding and flexibility than 40 years ago.

What is a sleeping problem?

Families have different expectations about what can be considered as a 'normal' sleeping routine for a young child. The ideal pattern is to have a child who settles quite easily at night and who sleeps the whole night through. In fact, all children (and adults) do wake during the night, but they simply settle themselves back to sleep without being aware of doing so. However, it is important to remember that many children do continue to wake occasionally for several years, and that some children will take a long time to settle themselves fully, depending on their temperament.

Sleeping problems tend to consist of two different patterns: difficulties in settling to sleep in the first place or waking frequently at night, or both. These patterns become a problem when they are persistent and when they have a marked impact on either you or your child. If your child's sleep pattern is so interrupted that he or she is always tired and grumpy the next day, then it is a problem. If your sleep is so interrupted that you are finding it hard to cope during the day on a regular basis then it is a problem.

How are sleep problems usually treated?

In theory, sleep problems are relatively easy to change for many children. Many health visitors run 'sleep clinics' and these usually focus on changing the habits of both the child and the mother to reduce the sleep problem. But some of the principles of sleep programmes are hard to apply to children with eczema. Some changes have to be made to apply a sleep programme to a child with eczema and sometimes it can be impossible to use the same principles as you would with a child with no eczema.

Most sleep programmes are based on 'behavioural principles'. It is assumed that the baby or child has 'learned' poor sleep habits and that the mother's response to the difficulties has (unintentionally) 'allowed' the sleep pattern to become established. A typical example is of a young child who has always had her mother present to settle her to sleep, and who has therefore learned that she 'needs' her mother there to fall asleep. So if the child wakes up at night she will call out to her mother and need her mother to come to her to enable her to settle again. If her mother doesn't come immediately, then the child gets more and more upset until the mother does come. The child's mother may try and resist her child's cries but after a few minutes feels that she should go to her child and settle her. The child responds to this by settling down, and after a while she does fall asleep again.

So the child becomes more and more convinced that she can only fall asleep with her mother there, and the mother becomes more and more convinced too. But she also feels it is not worth leaving the child to cry because she will end up getting less sleep than if she had responded straight away. The pattern continues and so neither the child nor the mother ever have the opportunity to learn that actually the child could learn to settle herself.

The treatment plan for this would involve helping the child to 'relearn' how to fall asleep without the help of her mother. A technique called 'controlled crying' is often used. There are different ways of doing this but the hard part is that the child does have to be left to settle herself even though she becomes quite upset about being left on her own. At first, the child is very reluctant to do this and will carry on crying and screaming to try and persuade her mother to come in, as she has done every day until now. The mother has to be very firm and leave the child for gradually increasing amounts of time. She may start by leaving her for first 3 minutes, then 5 minutes, then 7, etc. After the allotted time, when she does go in it has to be a brief visit to say to the child something like, 'I'm still here but you have to settle yourself', and not get persuaded by her pleading child. She then goes out and this time leaves the child a little longer than the time before. It is not unusual for young children to scream for a long time the first night – an hour or even more. However, if you can stick to it, then the next night it will reduce and by the fourth or fifth night it may be down to just five minutes. It is hard to believe that this is true, but it really does work like this. But as you can see you do have to be very determined to see it through. If you give in, you have to start right from the beginning again because you have probably made it worse by demonstrating to your child that he or she only has to keep screaming for long enough and you will go to him or her.

Can you use a sleep programme for a child with eczema?

There are a lot of difficulties in applying a sleep programme with a child with eczema. First of all, the child is often more uncomfortable than a child with healthy skin and it is therefore much harder for him or her to settle. Because of this, the child and family are more 'at risk' of developing settling difficulties than other families. A child with eczema can start off having 'genuine' difficulties with settling and sleeping comfortably through the night, and then develop poor sleeping habits in addition to this. If you accept that your child has greater difficulty than other children with settling and sleep, but try and deal with these as calmly and consistently as possible, you will reduce the chance of them developing 'behavioural sleep problems' in addition to their 'eczema sleep problems'.

Secondly, most mothers and fathers hate hearing or seeing their child scratch, and can't bear knowing how much damage the child may do to their skin if left to their own devices. Hearing your child scratching away at night and knowing that he or she is damaging his or her skin, can be hard to tolerate. It often feels so hard that it seems a lot easier to go to your child and try and help them to settle rather than to take the risk they will end up in a 'scratching frenzy'. You may reach a point of exhaustion when you can no longer do this and can put your head under the pillow to ignore your child's cries and scratching, but you have to be quite exhausted to do this. More likely, you will go to your child but will feel an enormous amount of tiredness and frustration, which makes it hard to help your child to settle. Obviously you can help them more if you are calm and reasonable. But it is not easy to be calm and reasonable when you are tired and have been woken up for the third time that night.

Although the behavioural principles on which sleep programmes are based are well established and based on sound theory, they do not take into account the complexity of our feelings towards our babies and children and they are a bit of an oversimplification of how sleeping problems develop. For example, if you yourself had a very strict mother who tended to ignore your tears or was not very comforting when you were upset, this may influence how you react to your own baby. Many parents try and compensate for what they see as the negatives in their own childhood; so they try and do things differently with their own children. In this example, the mother would probably respond very quickly and try to be very loving and responsive. So the way you feel about your role as the child's carer will influence how you respond to sleep difficulties.

However, we have also all learnt most of our parenting skills from our own experience of being parented. Parenting is the most important and difficult job you will ever have; but it is also the one for which you have the least training. It can be difficult to know ways to react other than the ones that you yourself have experienced. So we may also repeat the pattern of parenting we ourselves experienced because we do not know what other alternatives are possible.

This helps explain why sleeping programmes are very successful when they are carried out consistently, but also why a lot of parents simply find them too hard to carry through and abandon them before they have a chance to be successful. Or some parents decide they would rather put up with the sleep problem, than even try and tackle it, because it can appear quite a tough way to treat a young child. Your decision has to be based on how much the sleep deprivation does affect you and your child. Most children who are sleeping poorly are affected during the day and may be more grumpy and irritable. Most parents who are not getting enough sleep are also affected in the day and find it harder to tackle the normal difficulties that do come up. It is not easy to tackle a sleep problem; but it is not easy to live with the consequences of not tackling it either.

How do I start?

One helpful way to start is to try and identify for yourself what the difficult times are and how you may be influencing your child's sleep pattern. The aim is to try and separate out the sleeping problems that really are due just to the discomfort caused by eczema (eczema sleep problems) from those caused by bad habits (behavioural sleep problems). The poor sleeping habits will almost certainly have developed out of a combination of your child's difficulties settling and your own inconsistent way of managing sleep problems due to exhaustion and having to manage your child in difficult circumstances.

This involves keeping a sleep diary with a record of your child's sleep pattern and your response. This is not easy, because it all needs to be done at night and you are probably just keen to get back to bed. However, if you stick the diary on your child's bedroom door with a pen there too, you can just do it as you are going back to your room, without too much effort.

Box 5.	Example of a sleep diary.

Time	What child did	What I did
10:30–10:40	Woke up, hot and scratching	Gave her drink of cool water, opened window
11:45–12:30	Woke up, scratching arms	Put cream on and sat with her to help her to calm down
3:30–4:15	Came into our room, upset because couldn't settle	Initially took her into our bed. She kept us awake squirming. Took her back to her room and put more cream on
5:45–5:50	Came back into our room	Ended up with her in our bed and me in hers
7:00	All woke up when alarm went off	

Looking at this diary, there are elements of both an 'eczema sleep problem' and a 'behavioural sleep problem'. The first two times the child woke up was due to discomfort, but it may have been possible to prevent the second waking by putting cream on straight away the first time.

However, later in the night, the mother (understandably!) does respond inconsistently by first allowing the child into her bed, then taking her back to her room, and then, when the child comes back in again, giving up and going to sleep in the child's room. This is the type of waking that can probably be managed more effectively by some determination and energy put into planning how to manage the night waking. Although in the short term it does require more effort, it may pay off in the long run.

The advantage of keeping a diary is that it sometimes helps you to feel more committed to trying out a new way of managing your child's sleep. You may feel you know already what the patterns are, but somehow seeing it written down can improve your resolve and you might see patterns of which you had not been aware. It also helps you to become aware of how much your child is waking due to being uncomfortable, and how much has become a habit that you could try and tackle.

What sort of sleep programme is suitable for a child with eczema?

You have to be realistic when tackling a sleep problem with a child with eczema. It is unlikely that you will manage to get rid of sleep difficulties altogether, but you should be able to reduce them, and to introduce better habits for when (hopefully) your child's eczema does improve. Start with trying to tackle the problems caused by physical discomfort, the 'eczema sleep problems'. If you can improve your child's comfort you will improve their sleep. Then move on to the 'behavioural sleep problems', the bad habits that have developed because of the discomfort.

Step one

Is there anything I can do to improve the physical comfort for my child?

For a child with eczema the first thing is to be sure they are as physically comfortable as possible. This will improve their chances of settling themselves and reduce the chances of them waking up during the night.

- It is essential to get good control of the temperature in your child's bedroom. Ideally it is best to have a thermostat for this room or to have one fitted on the radiator in the room, and to ensure you have good enough ventilation in the room. All the child's sheets should ideally be cotton, as this seems to be non-irritant and to help to maintain a steady temperature. Have layers of bedding if possible because then it is easier to vary the amount of bedding depending on the external temperature.
- There are several companies that manufacture pyjamas that are adapted for children with eczema (see 'Useful addresses and contacts' at the back of the book) and these should be cotton, have non-irritant seams and, if necessary, have mitts and feet to reduce scratching.
- If possible, try and reduce the number of distractions and noises that might make it harder for your child to settle. This is not always easy if you have

other children sharing the room or the room is next to the toilet, etc.
However, it makes it a lot easier for the child to settle if they are not disturbed.

- Above all, establish a clear bedtime routine and try to stick to it as
consistently as possible. This should include bathing and applying their
moisturisers and, if necessary, other treatments. Check that you really are
using the treatment to maximum benefit at night. Gradually, decrease the
level of activity and include a quiet time just before settling. This will get
your child in the right frame of mind for sleep and will help to make it clear to
them that you are determined to get them to settle.

Step two

How can I help my child settle?

The most important way of helping a child to settle is to find some sort of routine
that suits both of you and that signals to the child that this really is bedtime. It
can be hard to establish and stick to a routine for settling because you yourself
are more tired and less patient at the end of the day. It is worth developing a good
sleep routine right from the beginning because habits develop early and are hard
to change once they are established.

What you are trying to do is to help your child to learn that they can
settle without you and that you are not ignoring their discomfort. If they are
uncomfortable, then you can help soothe them, but try and leave them before they
actually fall asleep so that they are settling on their own. Some parents find that
a 'massage' routine is helpful and that, as long as you keep this brief (and don't
expand it every time your child demands it), this is a helpful settling technique.
Choose whatever sort of massage that you feel comfortable with and that suits
your child. If their skin is too uncomfortable you can try massaging their head
or feet.

Other ways that parents use include putting on a lullaby or story tape, or a
night-light. But don't fall into the trap of putting the tape on again and again.

Antihistamines are often prescribed for children with eczema and they can
have a useful sedative effect. They can be extremely useful for managing sleep
problems for children with eczema but, as with all drugs, it is important to use
them properly. Try, if at all possible, to use them only when necessary, because
they do seem to become less effective over time. If you feel your child is not
responding any more to the type you are using, it is worth trying a different
type. The older antihistamines are actually much more effective than the newer
ones, precisely because they do have a sedative effect. Give the antihistamine
to your child at least half an hour before going to bed in order to maximise
the benefit.

How can I help my child get back to sleep once they have woken up?

The most important thing is to try and keep calm yourself and to give them the minimum amount of comfort to soothe their physical discomfort. (See Chapter 4 for more information on staying calm.) Try to avoid any sort of 'games playing' and avoid endless negotiation. Be kind but firm. If you develop a routine with a clear ending your child will learn that this is the signal for them to settle and that you are going to leave them to sleep again.

If your child is not particularly itchy and does not seem physically uncomfortable, then you can leave them to cry and use the 'controlled crying technique' described above.

- You have to be confident that you really can leave them and not give in part way through; but if you feel you can leave them, then do.

- Start by leaving them to cry for a short time, say 5 minutes. Then go in and just briefly check them and say that you are going to leave them to go to sleep. Try to be clear but firm and don't get caught up with any pleading or negotiating.

- Go out and leave them this time for a few more minutes, about 7 minutes. Again go in and just briefly let your child know you are still around but want them to go to sleep.

- Next time leave them for an additional 2 minutes, in total 9 minutes.

- Keep repeating this until your child does eventually fall asleep.

Be warned that the first night it can take a child an hour or more to settle. However, by the next night it will have reduced to about half this, and within a week it should be down to a few minutes only. This does involve quite a lot of determination on your part and parents often stop this halfway through because they think it is cruel to leave a child to cry for so long. However, if you do stick at it, it really does work quite quickly and your child will probably be just as bright and cheerful in the morning and will not appear traumatised by the night before.

If your child wakes up very itchy and uncomfortable you will have to do a bit of physical soothing to help them to settle. Have some moisturiser ready near their bed and calmly and soothingly apply it and give your child some encouragement. If the child has become very distressed and is seriously working up into a scratching frenzy then take them out of their bed or cot and help them calm down. It is not worth trying to reason with them at this point and it is certainly not worth getting into any form of argument or negotiation.

Being woken repeatedly at night can make parents feel quite desperate at times. If you feel you are about to 'lose it' then don't go into the room until you have calmed yourself down. The relaxation and hypnosis techniques we use for children can be very helpful for adults too, especially in the middle of the night. If you end up going in and shouting or acting in a punitive way this will almost certainly make your child feel worse. Wait until you are calm enough yourself before you try and manage your hysterical child. In Chapter 4 there are some suggestions for finding ways to help you to 'calm down'.

Make sure you agree some ground rules with your partner and stick to them. Don't switch tactics in the middle of the night. For example, make an active decision beforehand about whether or not you are going to let your child sleep in your bed with you. If you have decided that you are not going to let your child sleep in your bed, then stick to it. This is not easy – most of us will give in when we feel tired and will often opt for the easy option in the short term rather than the option that is best in the long term.

If you do not feel you can try the controlled crying technique, or if you feel there is little you can do to improve your child's comfort at night, then you may have to find a way of living despite having a child with a disrupted sleep pattern. It is probably worth trying to find creative ways of getting additional sleep occasionally, or at least organising your time so you can get a break. If you have a partner, negotiate some way that you can have some protected time for yourself; even the odd hour can make you feel a bit refreshed. Again, don't turn down offers of help, and try to think of the best way that it will be of help to you.

CASE STUDY CASE STUDY CASE STUDY CASE STUDY

Imran

Imran developed eczema when he was about 3 months old. He was quite an unsettled baby and because he was the third child his mother often felt she was so busy that Imran had to fit in around the family routine, rather than having his own bedtime routine. He did not find it easy to settle to sleep during the night and, because she was tired and did not want her older children to be disturbed by Imran, he frequently started off in his cot but ended up in his parents' bed. When her other children had gone to sleep in the evening, Imran would often still be awake and stay down with his parents until he dropped off to sleep.

Imran's mother felt constantly tired because of the broken nights, but also felt that she did not have any energy to try anything different. However, when they came back from a holiday when ▶

Imran was about $2\frac{1}{2}$ years old, Imran refused to sleep in his own cot and would scream until his mother moved him to her bed. He ended up staying every night in her bed and consequently his mother frequently slept badly because he was so restless at night. Although Imran's eczema was still quite extensive, it was clear that quite often he woke up more out of habit than because of itching.

Having spoken to her health visitor, Imran's mother decided that she had to try and tackle his sleeping problem because, even though he was getting older, she still never got a full night's sleep. She decided to start by tackling his settling problems and then the waking during the night.

Imran's mother started by rearranging the bedrooms so that Imran's brother (who usually shared his room) moved into his older sister's bedroom for a while. Then she started introducing a bedtime routine for Imran, by taking him into his own room after bathtime and reading him some books in there. She then put him down and sat with him for a few minutes while he had a musical box on. She then left the bedroom telling Imran that she was going to leave him to settle to sleep. She followed the controlled crying pattern as described above, but found the first three nights extremely hard. On the first night Imran cried for over an hour and although she did keep going in to check him he found it very hard to settle. The next night he still cried for about 45 minutes and the third night for 40 minutes.

However, he then began settling after just 15 minutes and, by the end of the second week, he fell asleep himself without any crying. During the night he did continue to wake up but he settled more quickly then, falling asleep after just 20 minutes or so.

Imran's mother was delighted with the improvement and continued his settling routine. However, when Imran's eczema flared up only two months later, she found she had to go to him again in the night because he was so itchy. His sleep pattern soon ▶

reverted to its previous pattern during the night, although Imran was still able to settle quite quickly when first going to sleep. It took another month for his skin to improve sufficiently for her to try leaving him to settle again. Again this was very hard, but in fact Imran's crying did not last as long this second time, and he began to go back to sleep on his own after just one week.

Although Imran did now sleep through about three nights in the week, he still woke occasionally during the other nights. However, his mother was now able to get some nights of uninterrupted sleep which helped her to feel much less irritable and encouraged her to continue with his routine. His sleeping pattern did get worse when his skin was particularly itchy, but when his skin improved his mother made sure that she kept up the settling routine to improve his sleep pattern.

Summary

- Sleeping problems are common in young children.

- Children with eczema often have disrupted sleep patterns.

- Sleeping problems cause a lot of distress for parents and children.

- Some sleeping difficulties are due to the discomfort caused by eczema; but some sleeping difficulties are due to 'bad habits' developing as a consequence of the child's discomfort.

- Behavioural methods for improving sleep patterns can be used for some children with eczema, with some modifications.

Understanding and managing diet for your child with eczema

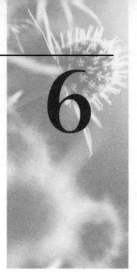

6

“It's a bit of a nightmare anyway with the food side of it. If she goes to parties you can't be there to see what she can and can't eat and in a way it's difficult for her, because obviously the other children they don't understand. And she looks like she's separated from the others all the time with the food she can't eat.”

“I was firm and said I wanted to try the dietary thing. It didn't do anything, but at least we knew we'd tried it properly.”

“I thought at one stage it might have been the cow's milk because it happened at a year old and that is when we put her on cow's milk. But I've tried her on goat's milk and it hasn't had much impact.”

There is so much controversy surrounding the question of whether or not eczema is related to diet. On the one hand, many children with eczema are on restricted diets at some point, but on the other hand, most doctors actively discourage the use of restricted diets.

When the evidence from very strictly controlled research studies of diet is considered, the evidence for the use of a restricted diet is not very encouraging. The conclusion drawn in the systematic review of treatments that was carried out recently is that 'there is little evidence to support an egg and milk free diet in unselected atopic eczema patients'. This is based on a review of all the published trials of dietary restriction. However, one of the problems identified in the review is that the quality of the studies is still quite poor and the existing studies are not conclusive *proof* that diet is not related to eczema either.

It is widely acknowledged that many parents of children with eczema do try a restricted diet at some point and that some complementary practitioners do advise trying diets that exclude some of the most common food allergens, for example milk, egg and wheat. However, it is extremely hard to stick to a restricted diet all the time, and many parents who try exclusion diets do not do so in a 'fair' way that would allow them to know whether or not the diet is successful. Unless you do stick to the restrictions consistently all the time, it will not be possible for you to know whether the diet is working or not. And it is extremely difficult to be consistent all the time, because so much of the processed food we do eat has added ingredients, such as milk powder. Unless you are prepared to read the ingredients lists of everything your child eats, it will be extremely hard to completely exclude all milk products. One of the reasons it has been so hard for research trials to produce conclusive evidence about the role of diet in eczema has been because so many families find restricted diets hard to do in practice and have 'dropped out' of the research trials.

It is rare to be able to easily identify a food that is definitely making your child's eczema worse. It is always tempting to look for causes when your child's eczema flares up and so you might look back on what your child ate the day before and think 'Perhaps it was the pizza/sweets/cheese/chocolate she ate yesterday'. This will only be misleading because you have ignored the other foods your child may have also eaten and picked out one possible culprit in a very arbitrary way. In other words, we are more likely to identify foods that have been suggested to us as possible causes of eczema and ignore all the other foods our child ate.

Having said that, a small minority of children with eczema do have a food allergy that is easily identifiable and can be confirmed by laboratory tests. However, these are only a small minority and, because the allergy is so clear, it is relatively easy to work out what the allergen is and then to exclude it. These children develop an instant skin reaction within a few minutes of contact with the food and this is why it is not hard to work out what has caused the allergic reaction. Sometimes, these types of allergies can be quite dangerous, and they can lead to a condition known as anaphylaxis. These severe allergies may be easier to identify, but they do require careful management, because of the severity of the allergic response and the need to be very vigilant about which foods the child can eat.

Fortunately these types of true food allergies are very rare and it is not this sort of reaction to food that most people think is relevant for children with eczema. With eczema most people consider that the food might be aggravating the eczema in some way, and this is known as an intolerance or sensitivity rather than a true allergy. With this sort of intolerance, even if milk did make your child's eczema worse you would not expect to see an effect straight away. It would probably take up to a month for it to be clear whether or not the withdrawal of milk is really having an effect or not. You would not see a dramatic difference on a day-to-day basis depending on what your child had eaten the day before.

With a baby or young child you are likely to be in control of all the food he or she eats. However, as your child gets older, he or she will probably start eating at other people's houses more often and going to parties where you have less control over what he or she eats. If your child has a serious allergy, especially if he or she is at risk of anaphylaxis, you will of course have to ensure that the food he or she is given is safe for him or her. However, most children do not like being treated differently from their peers and want to be able to join in with their friends. You need to have a very good reason to single your child out and have them treated 'differently', because it is likely to make them more self-conscious about themselves. A serious allergy is a good enough reason; but some parents do restrict their child's diet without good reason and this is unfair on the child. It can also be extremely confusing if you are not consistent and make it hard for your child to put up with not being able to eat all the foods they like, if you 'bend' the rules in certain situations. A young child is not going to find it easy if you won't let him have chocolate most of the time, but then occasionally give in and let him eat it. It is much better to make it very clear one way or the other. Either he is allowed chocolate or he isn't – don't keep changing the rules.

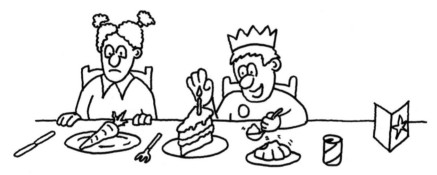

It can be hard for children on a restricted diet.

When is it appropriate to try a restricted diet?

It is generally thought that restricted diets are probably most effective with very young children and only for a small minority of children with eczema. Because of the lack of evidence that diet does make any difference, and the potentially very serious effects of restricting your child's diet, it is only worth trying an exclusion diet once you have given all the other forms of conventional treatment a really good trial. In other words, try all the other ways of treating your child's eczema first and consider a dietary approach only if these do not give you reasonable control. If you do want to try an exclusion diet, make sure you follow the method below, which I have called a 'fair trial', in order to find out whether or not the diet does make a real difference. The example below focuses on excluding cow's milk but can be adapted to any other form of exclusion.

Carrying out a fair trial of a restricted diet

You will need your doctor's help to carry out an exclusion diet, first to help you decide what to try and exclude and then also to prescribe any additional food supplements your child will need. Ask your doctor to refer you to a dietitian so that you can be sure that any diet you do try is safe for your child and is nutritionally adequate. She will also be able to advise you of all the different ways in which milk in particular, but also to a lesser extent egg or wheat may appear in a list of food ingredients in a disguised form. You need this information in order to be sure you are really giving the diet a fair trial. As discussed above, it is extremely hard to stick consistently to a restricted diet, especially if you are trying to withdraw a very common food substance such as milk, egg or wheat. For example, all of the following are a form of milk although this is not always known:

> whey, casein, skimmed milk powder, lactose, butter, milk protein, hydrolysed milk protein, buttermilk, yoghurt, cream, non-fat milk solids and cheese

In addition, in our diet, milk provides a very valuable source of protein, calcium and fat, all of which are essential components of a child's diet. If you just simply cut out milk without substituting other foods to provide adequate amounts of the above nutrients, then you may not be giving your child an adequate diet. So it is essential to get advice from a qualified dietitian to help ensure you are still giving your child an adequate diet.

You have to make sure you really do exclude the food from your child's diet and that you do it over a reasonable length of time so that you can be sure you will have picked up any effects. This means doing the diet for at least a month before deciding whether or not it has had any impact. Don't cheat – do it properly, otherwise you will be left with the constant uncertainty of whether the diet does really make any difference.

Try and enlist someone else as a 'witness' as to whether or not your child's eczema has improved. It is always difficult to tell from day to day whether his or her skin has improved because it can vary such a lot. If you ask your health visitor or your GP, or a dermatology nurse if you are attending an outpatient service, they could do a sketch of how extensive the eczema is and how red and inflamed the skin is before you start. There are some published scales for measuring the severity of eczema, and one of these would be ideal for this. After your child has been on the diet for four weeks, ask the same person to look at your child again and rate how severely affected your child is, using the same type of assessment, but without first looking back at the previous sketch. This is much better than just relying on your own judgement and it helps you to be sure that the diet really has made a difference.

Finally, whether or not there has been an improvement, you should then return to your child's normal diet, and include milk in their normal diet for another four weeks. Ask the same person to rate the severity again for you, without referring back to the first and second assessments, and then compare all three severity assessments. Eczema varies such a lot that some of the improvements seen following a new treatment are really only due to chance: they happened to coincide with the skin going through a good phase anyway. This is why it is important to reintroduce the milk again and to see if it does get worse again. If it doesn't, then it will probably not be worthwhile using a restricted diet because the improvement you initially saw was just most likely due to chance.

At the end of all this, you should have a good idea of whether or not the exclusion has made a worthwhile difference to your child's eczema. Although this is a lot of effort, unless you do the exclusion in this way you will never be able to be sure about whether you are doing the right thing for your child. It is worth putting this amount of investment in to find out whether a diet will help, because otherwise it is not really justifiable to keep your child on a restricted diet.

My doctor says that I shouldn't try a restricted diet because they don't work. Why won't he let me try this?

You may find that your doctor is extremely reluctant to let you try a dietary approach. This is because the evidence for using a dietary approach is so limited, and because the majority of people who do try dietary treatments do not do a 'fair trial' as described above. It requires a lot of commitment to stick to the fair trial and to stick to a restricted diet. Most families find that the practical difficulties make it difficult to be consistent and doctors have become alarmed by the casual way that some people restrict their child's diet without good reason – and, as we have seen, this can have an unnecessary physical and psychological impact on the child. If you talk to your doctor about doing a fair trial as described above, then you might be able to persuade him to let you have a go.

My 3-year-old child has bad eczema and his tummy does stick out and, although he eats really well, he seems have very frequent, loose stools. Is this as a result of a food allergy?

Many young children with bad eczema do seem to have this pattern of eating a lot and having loose stools. This is unlikely to be a form of allergy and it does usually improve as the child gets older. It is important to ensure that your child is growing and putting on weight as expected, and if he feels pain or a lot of discomfort in his tummy you should talk to your doctor about this. Most doctors think that these symptoms are linked to the skin condition and are a form of 'internal' eczema; however, this is poorly understood.

My 4-year-old is an extremely fussy eater and I am sure that her diet is very unhealthy. Is this making her eczema worse and how can I get her to eat a better balanced diet?

Food faddiness is very common indeed in this age group. This causes a lot of worry for parents because we know that a healthy diet is important for preventing some types of health problems in the long term and it is important to help children to manage to eat a healthy selection of foods, particularly fruit and vegetables. However, it is extremely unlikely to make eczema worse.

Mealtimes too often become a battleground for young children, and food ends up being used as a threat or a bribe or a means for expressing power. Force and excessive attention to faddy eating is nearly always counterproductive for young children. Some parents find themselves locked into a battle of wills with their child and the child is certain to win, because you cannot force your child to eat!

HELPFUL TIPS! HELPFUL TIPS! HELPFUL TIPS! HELPFUL

- The most important rule is to keep this problem in perspective. If your child is growing and eating a small range of foods, then try to relax and don't make it into more of a problem unnecessarily. It is very easy to forget many of the ways in which children manage to take in calories and nutrients and to underestimate what they are eating, so that it almost seems miraculous that they are gaining weight. Many children drink a lot of milk or juice in between meals, and these are both quite calorific.

- Keep giving your child very small amounts of food you want to encourage them to eat, such as a few slices of carrots, or one small sprig of broccoli, but don't nag them about it if they don't eat it. Every so often, say once a week, make sure you do include one food which is 'new' to their repertoire, but do this is in a very casual way and do not try and persuade them or bribe them to eat it. Just present it to them as an option and don't worry that they reject it. ▶

- Try and give everyone in the family the same meal and make the most of peer pressure by getting them all to sit down together as part of a normal routine. If you start cooking to order, as in a restaurant, your children will almost certainly make the most of this and there will be no incentive for them to even try foods they aren't familiar with or don't particularly like.

- If your child is not gaining weight, or is even losing weight, then you should seek further advice from your doctor or local child health clinic. Similarly, if you find your child is only eating sweet things, for example, just eating chocolate and drinking juice, you will need to get help because it will otherwise lead to serious dental problems.

CASE STUDY CASE STUDY CASE STUDY CASE STUDY

Daniel

Daniel was born 2 weeks after his due date following a healthy pregnancy. At about 12 weeks he began to develop an itchy rash, initially on his face and chest and then gradually spreading to cover most of his body area. The GP diagnosed eczema, and prescribed emollients and an antibiotic cream when it became infected.

Neither Daniel's mother or father had a history of eczema or asthma, and there was no family history of atopy. However, as Daniel got to 5 months his eczema had got so bad and so extensive that his mother tried a cow's milk free diet. Daniel had been exclusively breast-fed and his mother then excluded milk from her diet and weaned Daniel onto a cow's milk free diet. This did result in a improvement in Daniel's skin; however, Daniel's GP was not convinced that this was necessary and advised his mother to try introducing cow's milk rather than an alternative such as soya milk.

When Daniel was given his first bottle of cow's milk formula at age 7 months he had an immediate allergic reaction, with urticaria ▶

initially on his face and then spreading over his body. It was clear that it was an allergic reaction and this was agreed by his GP. A referral was made to the dietitian for further advice and Daniel was subsequently weaned onto soya milk. He continued to have mild eczema until he was about 18 months old and then it gradually disappeared.

He continued to have a milk allergy until he was about 7 years old and he was seen regularly at an allergy clinic to reassess this. It was also discovered that he was allergic to peanuts and to some tree nuts. Fortunately, his eczema completely resolved by the time he was 3 years old

Summary

- Many families do try a restricted diet for their child with eczema.

- Restricted food diets are most likely to be helpful for younger children.

- Only a small minority of children with eczema have a demonstrable food allergy and improve on a restricted diet.

- Restricted diets are hard to stick to consistently.

- It is important to give the restricted diet a fair trial in order to be sure whether or not it is effective.

- It can be both physically and psychologically harmful to put a child on a restricted diet if this is nutritionally inadequate or is unnecessary.

Managing teasing and improving your child's self-esteem

7

> **"**He gets called all sort of names – scabby, flaky, spotty. But I tell him that you've got to be brave and just rise above it and deal with it.**"**

> **"**I feel like shouting it in the playground, 'You can't catch it' – the intolerance of other people!**"**

One of the difficult aspects of having a skin problem is that it is visible to others. Unlike other types of childhood illnesses you therefore have to deal with other people's reactions all the time. At first, young children are not even consciously aware of the way other children or adults react to them. However, self-consciousness increases with age during childhood and by the time your child is an adolescent they will be acutely sensitive to how they are seen by other people. Fortunately many children do grow out of their eczema before adolescence, but this can be a particularly difficult time for someone with eczema.

As a society we place a lot of importance on appearance and we are surrounded by unrealistic images of 'perfect' beauty. For example, photographs of models are retouched to make their skin appear absolutely flawless and it is not possible for real people to ever achieve the sort of perfect skin that is shown on magazines. We are also not a very tolerant society and do not easily accept people who appear different. It is a difficult climate for a child with eczema to grow up feeling good about themselves.

Parents will also feel some of these pressures. It is hard not to feel sorry for your own child when he or she is next to another young child who has a 'peaches and cream' complexion and who appears so comfortable and confident in their own skin. Rather than getting all the positive comments that many other parents receive, such as 'She looks so gorgeous' or 'How smooth his skin is', you may have to deal with reactions of uncertainty and even physical revulsion from others. It is important to be able to help your child develop a positive and confident approach to managing the reactions of others, but this is hard to do when it still upsets you.

Dealing with curiosity and inquisitiveness in young children

Young children are very direct about their curiosity and about their immediate reaction to what they see. So young children will often ask very directly, 'What is wrong with his skin?' Or they may say something about their immediate reaction, 'Ugh, her skin's horrible. It's all wrinkly'. Young children react in this way because they haven't yet learned to modify their immediate response to fit in with the social situation. They are not doing it with any intention of hurting the other child.

The best way of dealing with these types of reaction is firstly to tell them the facts, for example:

> ❝She's got eczema. It's a type of skin problem that makes her skin very dry. You can't catch it.❞

If appropriate, you can then say something about how hurtful those sorts of remarks can be. It is important not to do this in an angry or blaming way, because you have to assume that the child who made the comment was only doing it out of an immediate reaction rather than any desire to hurt. Rather than blaming them for saying this, you are trying to educate them about how their reaction affects your child. For example you could say:

> ❝She doesn't like it when other people stare at her/say things that might hurt her feelings – so please try not to say those sort of things to her.❞

Dealing with curiosity and inquisitiveness in adults

You may also find that adults stare at your child or, more subtly, take a good look at your child without actually saying anything. You have to find your own style for dealing with these looks, and you may find you can use different approaches depending on the situation. Some strategies include, giving them the information and showing you understand their curiosity.

> ❝You are obviously wondering what's wrong with his skin. Its actually eczema, so it's not catching.❞

If you feel up to it you can try using humour or just chat to the other person about other things.

Try not to get too negative about these reactions. They are mostly due to curiosity and uncertainty about how to deal with the situation rather than maliciousness.

What is the best way to deal with teasing and name-calling?

Most children with eczema experience some episodes of being called names and being teased about their skin. Although this may not appear a major problem, because it is 'only' name calling or teasing, it can eat away at a child's self-confidence if it happens to them frequently. Some name-calling and teasing will happen to every child at some point, but when it is persistent or severe it is a form of bullying and no child should be treated in this way.

It is important for you to talk to your child about name-calling and teasing because children often feel very reluctant to talk about being teased and may not want to bring it up themselves. They may be worried that you will confront the other child and make the situation worse. They may be trying to minimise the problem because it might upset you or because they find it too upsetting themselves. Help them to develop a less emotional response to this inevitable teasing by explaining that sometimes people find it hard to accept people who look different, but that any reasonable person knows that it is what is inside that it is really important. Try to discourage aggressive responses and help your child develop more assertive responses instead. Try not to become over-emotional yourself when talking to your child and don't keep on and on bringing it up, even if you are thinking about it a lot. Your child should not have to deal with your difficulties as well as his or her own!

Teasing can come in different forms and the intention behind the teasing determines the best way of dealing with it. For example, young children may say quite hurtful things quite innocently, with no intention of hurting. They say things out of curiosity or impulsiveness. On the other hand, older children can be very cruel on purpose. They may say or do things deliberately to hurt other children, although this is usually done in a very crude and explicit way. Adults also tease and bully, but they are much more sophisticated in the way that they do this. Sometimes older children or adults act in a way that is inconsiderate or thoughtless, but they do not actually intend to hurt someone else – they just haven't thought through the way their behaviour will affect the other person.

Teasing and bullying have always existed in any group setting. However, most schools have had to become much more open about their policy towards bullies and bullying is tackled in a far more direct way than in the past. For example, all schools should now have a written anti-bullying policy. However, despite this openness about how unacceptable bullying is, it is still hard for them to deal with the sort of experience of a child with eczema, which is often worse than 'normal' teasing but may not be as severe as 'bullying'. After all, every child will experience some level of teasing – it might be about their name, their hair colour or the clothes they wear. They will get teased about something at some point. However, it becomes a problem for children who experience this a lot of the time, or where the teasing becomes a way to exclude the child from a group, or when it is so common that it makes them feel like a victim.

My child is being teased occasionally at school. How seriously should I take it?

Like any other child, your child will need to learn some ways of managing group situations, including the natural competitiveness that comes of being part of a group. You can't, and shouldn't try, to protect them from this. However, you may need to help them to find ways to tackle teasing or name-calling about their eczema and help them to develop some standard phrases they can repeat themselves as they get older. Your aim is to try and reduce the likelihood of the teasing becoming entrenched to avoid your child feeling like, and being seen as, a victim. But you also want to be able to develop your child's own sense of self-worth, so that he or she does feel good about dealing with other people.

There are some classic phrases designed to be quick retorts that help the child feel they have got something to say back immediately. They can be useful because they give the child an 'automatic' response in a fraught situation – for example, 'Sticks and stones may break my bones but names can never hurt me' or 'What you say is what you are'.

The problem with these sorts of phrases is that they are quite likely to lead to escalation of name-calling rather than defusing the situation. They can be said in a very aggressive way and even if they are not said aggressively, they can be perceived as aggressive. This is then more likely to make the other child respond again – if not this time, then later.

It is better to teach your child to use similar phrases but to say them to him or herself as a form of positive self-talk. For example, teach them phrases like 'It is what is on the inside that counts' or 'I'm worth ten of them'. This is not easy for a child to do for himself at first; you will have to adopt this way of managing comments yourself as an example for your child to learn from. This will mean you literally having to say this to your child when you are able to, and to explain to them that it is useful to have a few things to say back quickly in situations like these.

You can also teach your child 'exit' strategies, that is, ways of helping them to get out of difficult situation. Although we often advise children to 'just ignore it' it can be a lot more helpful to help them find something *active* to do rather than expecting them to take the passive role of ignoring comments. The reason ignoring is seen as a useful strategy is because it prevents the other child from gaining satisfaction out of 'winding up' the victim, which could lead to an increase in teasing. However, by getting out of the situation your child is both protecting him or herself and very clearly giving the message that they are not a victim who will passively absorb any amount of name-calling. If she is able to walk away with dignity and purpose it reduces the effect of being called names.

It is often said that children who bully have been bullied in the past and this is the only way they know how to behave with other children. Whilst this may be true for some children, many children tease or bully because they simply don't think about the consequences, or because they fail to appreciate the impact of the teasing/ bullying on the other child. Once these are clearly demonstrated to them, they do feel remorse and will learn from this. This is where the culture in the school can be so important. Schools that teach their pupils to respect one another from the very beginning help the children to develop what is sometimes called 'emotional literacy'. This is relevant to all forms of difference that the children will come across in the school: gender, race, appearance, etc. This approach helps children to think explicitly about how other children feel and to understand the impact of their own behaviour on others. The culture then develops of behaving in a considerate and thoughtful way towards all other people.

However, there are some children who appear to enjoy some of the social power that they get as a result of teasing and bullying other pupils. In effect, these children begin to realise that they can manipulate other people for their own purposes. Recent studies of these types of bullies suggest that they do not do this just because they do not know how to behave with other children or because they do not understand it might hurt another child. They do it precisely because they are able to understand the usefulness and power of these techniques and understand the social status it gives them. It is no help at all to teach these children 'emotional literacy' because they already know – all too well – how to use social skills to their advantage. This sort of manipulation can be very subtle and damaging. This sort of persistent bullying or manipulation can only be addressed by getting the child's teacher to address the problem, and by using very direct sanctions for any teasing or bullying. If your child is being picked on by one these types of bullies you should not expect your child to have to manage it alone – a much more active approach is needed.

What should I do if my child is being bullied?

If your child is being teased or bullied frequently at school, you need to enlist the help of his or her teacher. Most teachers will listen to your concerns and take them seriously, particularly if they are directly affecting your child's attendance at school or his or her wellbeing. What may appear as a minor problem to a teacher, however, can be a major problem for your child. It is important for you to be able to explain to the teacher what your child is experiencing, so it can be helpful to write down any comments your child has made or any particular observations you have made. Have a look at the school's anti-bullying policy and see if all the sanctions and strategies suggested there are being used.

Usually, class teachers are well aware of particular children who are causing difficulties for other pupils. However, they may have a limited number of resources and strategies to use. Agree a plan with the class teacher, and if the situation does not improve, write a letter to the school asking for a meeting to address your concerns. These sorts of meetings can be very daunting and very emotional for you, so take a friend or your partner along to help you out.

If the school needs help with thinking of useful strategies then the organisation Kidscape provides some excellent books and leaflets for schools, including some classroom exercises, that address bullying in schools. If the school does not know about this organisation, then give them their address (see 'Useful addresses and contacts' at the back of the book for details). If they do, then ask them which of the strategies they are going to put into place.

How can I improve my child's self-esteem?

In order to counterbalance the negative reactions your child may experience outside the family, it is essential to actively promote his or her self-esteem directly. A child feels loved and feels good about himself when he is praised often and when his efforts are valued as well as his successes. Show your child that he is lovely to you. Show him physically by lots of cuddles and affection, but tell him as well. We are not always very good at giving praise, and some parents find it uncomfortable, but children do thrive on it.

All children have strengths and your child will feel a lot better about himself if you encourage his strengths as well as just dealing with all the problems that occur. Help him experience success by finding out what his strengths are and doing some positive things together related to this. Help him to take part in 'show and tell' or circle time at school by encouraging him to take any certificates or particular achievements into class.

Even if your child's appearance is affected by eczema, you can still try and help him look his best. Help him to build up his sense of pride in himself by telling him he looks good in an outfit that does suit him. Help him develop his own sense of style so that he can feel pleased with himself and confident with others. Although many children, particularly boys, don't appear to very interested in clothes or shopping for clothes, they will probably respond to you picking up something special for them and telling them how good they look in it.

Get your child to recognise when he or she has done well and to acknowledge his own strengths. This does not mean making your child conceited or encouraging him to gloat about his achievements over other people, but he should give himself credit when he has done well, particularly when it was something that was quite challenging for him.

If your child is not very confident in social situations, you can help them to build up skills to deal with difficult situations. These are similar to the 'assertiveness' skills that are often taught to adults. For example, help them to stand tall and to make requests themselves, by speaking clearly and looking the other person in the eye. This may sound and feel uncomfortable at first but if you practise in front of a mirror you can show your child how different they look when they do behave

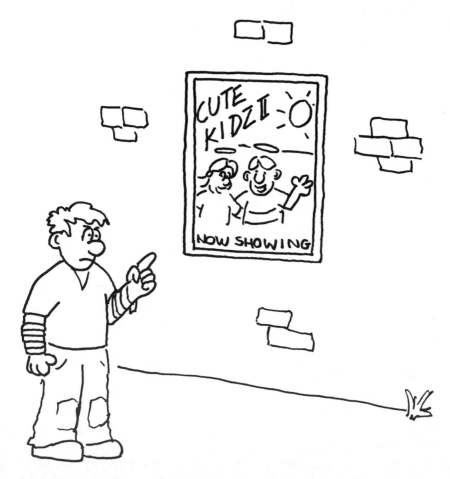

Our society overvalues physical beauty and it can be hard growing up looking different.

confidently. Try to do this in a 'matter-of-fact' way rather than becoming emotional about it, and do not force an unwilling child to do these sorts of exercises. But, even if they cringe at these suggestions now, they may take up the ideas at a later stage.

Your child will be bombarded with images of beauty from the outside world and will have to grow up in a culture that rates physical beauty (of a certain sort) very highly. However, we all know that physical beauty is not a guarantee of love and happiness and many, many people who are very successful are not conventionally beautiful. When opportunities arise, make sure you challenge the 'beauty culture' myth with your child. You can point out clear examples of people who have succeeded despite disabilities or talk about the shallowness of the beauty culture. Don't overdo this and become a complete bore, but make sure you always give your child this alternative view of success.

If your child becomes extremely self-conscious about their eczema, or if it is very disfiguring, then you might want to get further information and help from an organisation called Changing Faces. This charity helps children and adults with all forms of disfigurement and produces some excellent publications as well as running workshops for children and adults. See 'Useful addresses and contacts' at the back of the book for details of how to contact them.

My child is becoming aggressive too – how can I prevent this getting worse?

Unfortunately, some children who have been bullied or teased do become aggressive themselves. This is particularly unfortunate because, once a child does this, he or she is likely to lose any sympathy from other children or adults. Even if the aggressive behaviour is a direct consequence his or her own experience, this is more than likely to make the situation worse.

Be careful not to encourage any aggressive behaviour. At times it is all to easy to encourage an aggressive reaction, particularly when you feel fed up with your child being the one who is picked on or treated badly. Don't let yourself do this because, although it feels better in the short term, it will not help your child in the long term. It is important for your child not to be a victim and not to appear like a victim; but using physical violence himself or herself is not the answer.

There are other ways to build up your child's confidence so that he or she does not take up a victim stance. Build up his or her self-esteem as described above. Show him or her that you will not accept him or her being treated badly by taking action yourself with the school as suggested above.

If you find out your child has been bullying someone else, then try and find out what happened and talk to your child to help them to understand what they did was wrong. Once they have acknowledged they did something wrong, get them to apologise, either in person or writing. For example, get them to write a short apology to the other child or, if they are not able to write this on their own, then you write it and get them to sign it. Don't keep reminding them of the incident – once you have done the apology, start with a clean sheet and don't keep punishing them about it. Hopefully, they will not try this again.

I can't bear seeing my child being teased – I feel so angry and upset myself. I find I can't even talk to other people about it without bursting into tears. What should I do?

There will be days when you are unable to deal calmly with the looks or comments your child receives. At times you may act very aggressively yourself towards other adults staring or a teacher who does not seem to understand. These incidents usually happen when you are feeling particularly sensitive yourself. Maybe you are tired or worn out, or maybe you have been frustrated about something else and you take your temper out in this way. However, if you feel like this frequently, it is not helpful for your child to see you become so upset, defensive or aggressive.

We all have our own areas of sensitivity. If you yourself were teased as a young child you will long for things to be better for your own child. Seeing your own child hurt or upset can vividly bring back all the hurt you yourself experienced. However, you cannot fight your child's battles for them, it is important for them to do the learning directly rather than indirectly through you.

All parents feel upset themselves when their child is upset or hurt. However, it is important for you to find a way to deal with your upset that doesn't transmit your problems to your child. Allow yourself some time to think through why it upsets you so much, and talk about this to your partner or another member of your family or a friend, if possible. If you feel that you cannot handle it yourself with your friends and family, then you may be able to arrange to see a counsellor through your GP. Many surgeries offer counselling sessions, although these are in short supply so you might have to wait for an appointment.

CASE STUDY CASE STUDY CASE STUDY CASE STUDY

Samantha

Samantha had eczema since she was a baby. Although it was well controlled, her hands were one of the worst-affected areas and ▶

hence it was very visible. Samantha started school when she was nearly 5 years old. Her mother had explained to the school in advance about Samantha's eczema, because she often needed to have cream applied during the day.

Samantha had always been rather shy and had taken a while to settle at her nursery. However, she settled quite easily at school and become friendly with a few other children and was gaining in confidence. During the second half of the autumn term, Samantha's eczema got a bit worse and she appeared quite unsettled at school. On a few occasions she told her mother she felt sick and didn't eat breakfast, so her mother kept her off school. The third time this happened, her mother sent her in to school anyway, thinking that Samantha was beginning to avoid something at school and she arranged to meet with Samantha's teacher. Samantha's teacher was quite reassuring and said that, although Samantha was very quiet at school, she was 'no problem at all' and that this was just part of Samantha settling in at school.

However, one day on the way home from school, Samantha's mother heard another child shouting out 'There's scabby Samantha' and felt Samantha cringe. One of the boisterous boys from her class rushed up to Samantha and then spoke to her quite happily and normally and was very friendly to Samantha. Samantha's mother felt unsure how to deal with it then and there but asked Samantha about it later.

Samantha initially appeared quite reluctant to talk about it and told her mother it was nothing and said she quite liked this boy. However, her mother felt Samantha was not admitting to herself how much it upset her, and gently talked to Samantha a bit more about teasing and how it can hurt, even if the child is quite friendly as well. Samantha told her mother that several of the children now called her 'scabby Samantha' and that they didn't want to hold her hand or be her partner because of her hands. She tried to put a ▶

brave face on it and said that her best friend, Kelly, would often be her partner anyway, and that she knew the eczema wasn't catching.

The next day Samantha's mother arranged to meet with her teacher, and told her about the name-calling and problems which Samantha had reported. The teacher was sympathetic and helped to think of ways in which she could talk to the class in general about name-calling, as well as talking to the individual boy concerned. She arranged for the boy to sign a note to Samantha saying that he had not meant to hurt her feelings and would not do so again. Samantha's mother was given the note and at home talked to Samantha about how he had hurt her feelings and how he had now learned not to do this.

Samantha continued to be quite shy at school but her confidence grew over the year and she made some good friends. Her mother was pleased with the way the school had tackled the problem early on and encouraged Samantha to tell her if anything similar happened at school.

Summary

- Many children with eczema do experience name-calling and teasing.

- If the intention is not to hurt, then explain what eczema is and explain why it is hurtful to call children names.

- If it is intended to hurt, it is a form of bullying and it is important to act to prevent it getting worse.

- Improve your child's self-esteem directly by encouraging them and helping them develop their strengths.

- Challenge the 'beauty myth'.

Growing up with eczema

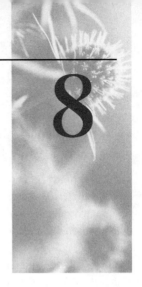

8

"Initially the doctor said she had atopic eczema, she'll grow out of it. When she was 1 year old, or 18 months, they said she'd grow out of it when she's four or five. Then it became five or six, then seven and its always got worse ... Maybe when she's a bit older, when she's in her teens she might grow out of it."

"You can feel guilty about it to a certain extent, but you just try to help them manage it and, maybe because I've had it for as long as I have, you know I do understand how he feels."

"I know it's just through her Dad that she's got it. It upsets him to know that he's passed it on to her ... He hates to see her when her skin's flared up."

When a baby or young child develops eczema, it is usually assumed that he or she will grow out of it. Most parents will be told that it is normal for the eczema to get better as the child grows older. This is true for children with eczema as a whole group, but it is still hard to predict for an individual child when, or even if, he or she will be free of eczema. Nonetheless, it is still a reassuring and encouraging fact that so many children do grow out of eczema and there is a good chance that even if the eczema remains, it will be much less severe than when the child was very young.

However, for some children, the eczema remains a chronic problem that does not resolve in the early childhood years, as had been expected, and at some point both the child and the parents have to learn to accept the eczema, rather than just hoping that it will gradually get better of its own accord. This brings with it a shift in thinking about the eczema, from hoping to find a 'cure' to managing the condition as well as possible. This final chapter explains some of the common questions and problems for parents with children whose eczema does not go away in early childhood.

My child has had eczema now for 4 years and it does not seem to be getting better. Should she be referred to a dermatologist?

The vast majority of children who have eczema are treated by their GP alone and do not get referred to a dermatologist. It is usually the children with chronic, severe eczema, whose skin has not responded well to the most common forms of treatment who do get referred on to a specialist. If your child's eczema does not seem to be improving or if your child's eczema often flares up and you do not feel you have good control over the symptoms, then it is worth asking your GP to refer him or her to a dermatologist, if this has not already been done, in order to consider whether further treatments would be appropriate.

As well as offering additional advice about the types of treatment your GP will have prescribed, there are additional specialist treatments that can only be offered by dermatologists, although some of these would only be offered to older children when all other treatments have been tried. In addition, some dermatology clinics have specialist dermatology nurses who can spend time with you, helping you to get the best from the treatments you are using, such as showing how to apply wet wrap bandages. It can be helpful to go through the details of your skin routine in order to think through whether you are using the treatments as effectively as possible, and to consider ways of making the routine more acceptable for you and your child.

There are also some very specialised treatments that are only used when all the other types of treatment have not been successful, and therefore tend to be used only for older children. These include PUVA, a treatment that involves taking an oral dose of a medicine called psoralen and receiving a form of radiation or light therapy. Some children might also be offered an immunosuppressant drug, such as cyclosporin. But these types of treatment require careful supervision and monitoring because of the potential for very serious side effects of the drugs used.

My child is due to start school and she still has quite bad eczema. How much help can I expect from the school?

First of all you need to have some discussion with the school about what your child's needs will be in school, preferably before your child starts so that it is all in place at the beginning. For example, does your child need to have emollient available during the daytime, and how will this be arranged with the school. Schools do have to keep most types of medical treatment safely locked away, but they should allow some flexibility for emollients. You will have to make sure that your child feels comfortable about putting the treatment on at school and if necessary arrange a room he or she can go to for some privacy.

Then you need to talk to your child's teacher regularly to make sure that you are dealing with any problems that might arise as a result of your child's eczema, before they become entrenched. This will probably include lots of practical issues, such as what to do if your child becomes too hot or itchy during the day, and how to manage days when your child is very tired because he or she has not slept well. But it might well include more emotional issues too, such as how the class should be told about his or her eczema and how to manage teasing or name-calling. You may need to give the school some information about eczema, because they may not be familiar with the particular needs of a child with eczema. The National Eczema Society produce some leaflets that can provide basic information for your school.

If your child's eczema is very severe then the school may want to put him on the register of children with 'special educational needs'. This sounds daunting but is actually a way of ensuring that children who do have additional medical or psychological needs can get the most from school, by giving them the extra facilities they need to ensure that they get access to the full curriculum. If necessary, a child can be given a 'Statement of Special Educational Needs', which defines their specific needs, and aims to identify ways of managing these needs. However, this is usually only done when the school has already tried to find ways of addressing the needs of the child themselves. It is unlikely that a child with eczema would need such a statement, because schools should be able to provide the extra input a child with eczema may need from their own resources.

My child is now 14 and is responsible for his own skin care routine. However, I don't think he is doing it well enough and his skin is just looking worse. He won't let me do the treatment any more, so what should I do?

At some point all children do have to take over their skin care routine from their parents. This is usually a gradual process: as the child becomes older he does a little bit more for himself, until finally he doesn't even want the parent to be involved any more.

However, as in many other areas of life, young adolescents are not as conscientious about taking care of themselves as their parents would like them to be. It can be hard as a parent to see that your child is not keeping up the treatment as well as he should. However, this is almost an inevitable stage that you have to go through as you gradually let go of the responsibility of caring for him and hand that over to the young person himself. It helps to remember that nearly all parents are better at looking after their children than they are at looking after themselves. So it is possible that your son will never take as much care of himself as you did of him when he was young, but he will probably take as good care of himself as you do of yourself.

You have to decide how much damage he is doing to himself as a result of not doing the treatment, and it is only if the damage is really significant that you should intervene. If his skin does get a bit worse, then hopefully he will realise the importance of a good skin care routine himself and, because of his own discomfort, he will try and improve his own routine. If this is all that will happen, then, even though it is difficult for you, you do have to let him learn this for himself.

If, however, you suspect he is feeling generally rather hopeless and fed up and his lack of skin care is actually a sign of feeling miserable or depressed, then you should try and help him through this. When adolescents do feel very low they can lose interest in taking care of themselves and hence this can be a sign of general low mood. Maybe he is having a particularly difficult time at school, or he is very unhappy about a situation at home. If he is reluctant to talk to you, it can be helpful for him to talk to another member of the family or a friend's parent. Some schools also employ counsellors who are trained to talk to young people who are feeling distressed. As you can probably remember from your own adolescence, many young people do experience quite marked mood changes, but most of these are entirely normal and part of the process of growing up. Occasionally, however, these mood changes become more severe and these young people do require more help.

My child's eczema does not seem to be getting better as predicted. I still feel this is unfair but I'm beginning to accept that he may have to learn to live with eczema. How can I help him do this?

If you have reached the point of realising that your child is going to have to manage to live with eczema, then it is important to develop a positive approach to tackling the condition. There is enormous variation in the way that children respond to the additional demands placed on them as a result of having a chronic physical illness, and the way a child adapts is closely related to the sort of support their family has been able to provide. There is no doubt that both the child and his or her family do have to cope with a higher level of demand or stress than a family of a healthy child, and this does mean both the child and family are at higher risk of developing difficulties as a result of this. But some children are very resilient and find ways of minimising the impact of the condition on themselves, and they are helped a lot in this by the attitude of their family.

Developing a positive approach to living with eczema

- Acknowledge the impact of eczema.
  The first step in developing a positive approach to eczema is to be able to acknowledge the impact of the condition and of the treatment. This means

accepting that, despite all your attempts to find the reason for the condition, there may well be no definitive cause to account for the eczema. If you continue to harbour unrealistic hopes about a 'cure' that is just around the corner you will never accept the limitations of the condition. This does not mean that you have to give up trying any new treatments, but it does mean that you have to develop a critical view of these and have realistic expectations when you do take something new on.

- Deal with any guilt or anger about the cause of the eczema.
The next step is to be realistic about why it is your child has eczema and to try to deal with any feelings of guilt or blame you have towards yourself, your partner, or even your child with eczema. There is a genetic component to eczema and therefore it is quite common that one parent has a strong family history of atopic conditions, and he or she can end up feeling very guilty about being the partner who has 'caused' the child's eczema. This can lead to a number of difficult situations. If there are difficulties in the parent's relationship anyway, this guilt can become part of a cycle of blame, particularly if the partner who has no history of eczema is already feeling resentful about the amount of caring they have to do. They may well blame their partner for all the difficulties they are now experiencing and even say this to them at times.

On the other hand, it can be useful if one of the parents had bad eczema as a child and can understand and anticipate some of the difficulties that may arise. Although the child's experience is likely to be different in some ways, it may well be that some of the parent's own experience could be helpful for the child.

It is also possible for problems to be minimised by other members of the family if there is a strong history of eczema. If you are finding it hard to cope, you may have to put up with other people saying it is 'only' eczema or implying that you are making a mountain out of a molehill. You may find that unfair comparisons are made between how 'easy' things are now compared to in the past, and this can make you feel very inadequate. It can be helpful to remember that we do have different expectations now of treatments and of the sort of help we are entitled to when we have a child with a medical condition. In addition, it is very easy to look back at an experience that you have been through and to 'forget' how hard it was at the time, simply because you have now survived – so it doesn't seem as difficult now as it was at the time.

If you do have strong feelings of anger or guilt about your child's eczema, this is certain to make it harder for you to manage your own child's difficulties calmly. It is important for you to be able to move on from this, and most people find that this is best done by first recognising the problem and then being able to talk it through with someone you trust. In the first instance, this can be a good friend or a relative who you think will understand. Alternatively, you may get the opportunity to talk it through with one of the health care team involved in your child's care. It can be difficult to find time for this sort of conversation, so it is sometimes not possible in a normal clinic situation. It is often most helpful to talk to someone who understands eczema well, so you may find it most helpful to meet someone through your local branch of the National Eczema Society. However, if you feel that you need more help than this, then your GP can refer you to a counsellor or a psychologist who can help you think through the issues you find hard. Although it is hard to make time for yourself to do this, it may often help to tackle these sorts of problems early on both for your child's sake and for your own.

- Be realistic about the demands of the treatment and how well you are actually doing it.
  This means being realistic about what you can achieve and being honest with yourself about how well you do manage the treatment. This does not mean being critical of yourself because you find it frustrating to manage your child's skin care. Rather, it means accepting that it is a frustrating form of treatment and that you do have to do it repeatedly. Every so often you probably do need to 'refresh' your routine and think through whether there are any ways you can improve it. If you have let the routine slip for a while, this should help you to begin again with renewed commitment.

- Expect some ups and downs.
  It is extremely likely that the physical severity of your child's eczema will vary over time. In addition, there will be times when the eczema causes particular difficulties and at these times your child may feel cross or frustrated by the demands placed on them because of the eczema. For example, when your child first goes away for several nights on his or her own, and has to manage their skin routine independently, they may well resent having to manage these additional responsibilities compared to their friends. These times will be hard for you as a parent too, because as well as coping with this sort of transition (which all parents have to manage) you will have the additional worry of ensuring your child can manage the treatment and any particularly difficult situations on their own. However, there will probably also be times when you are managing quite well and the eczema is quite settled. Try and appreciate these while they last. Also recognise that chronic eczema varies over time and these ups and down are part of its normal course.

- Keep a sense of perspective.
  Many children with chronic eczema (and other physical illnesses) do have to put up with more than their healthy peers. They do experience some

physical discomfort, and have to tolerate repetitive treatment regimes, and they may be subjected to teasing and some difficulties with peers. However, some of these children do show remarkable resilience and strengths, and often appear to be more considerate and caring than their healthy peers. Children who experience chronic physical illnesses often do become more tolerant with other people because of their own experience, and this is a very positive quality. It is easy to forget all the positives and all the things your child does well, and to focus only on the negatives. It is important to keep a sense of perspective and to make sure that you still recognise all the normal things your child can do, rather than just focusing on the things they find hard. This will help them to think positively about their abilities too and not to let the eczema take over their life. This does not mean denying the undoubted restrictions that they also have, but it does mean keeping these difficulties in perspective.

Some parents also feel that, despite all the difficulties of caring for a child with eczema, they themselves do gain some benefits from their experience. For example, many parents become very active members or fundraisers for the National Eczema Society, or go on to act as volunteer local contacts, who can talk to other parents of children with eczema. Many parents also become real experts in this field and end up as well-informed as health professionals. Whilst it would be misleading to think that these small gains compensate for some of the difficulties experienced, it is important to remember that are some positive aspects to be gained from caring for a child with eczema.

Summary

- Eczema does improve over time for most children, but it is very frustrating for the minority of children whose eczema does not improve.

- Develop a positive attitude towards managing eczema to help your child cope with their eczema.

- Allow them to take over the care of their skin as they grow older.

- Keep a sense of perspective and notice when things go well.

Useful addresses and contacts

General

The National Eczema Society
Hill House
Highgate Hill
London N19 5NA
Tel: 020 7281 3553
Eczema Information Line: 0870 241 3604
www.eczema.org

This is the main charity working with people with eczema in the UK. It produces a regular magazine and a series of extremely helpful factsheets about aspects of eczema. It also promotes research into the causes of and treatments for eczema and helps to raise public awareness of the needs of people with eczema. It also has a network of local volunteer contacts and support groups run by people with experience of eczema.

www.eczemavoice.com

This is a website started by people with eczema which contains information and helpful hints and tips from people with eczema.

Disfigurement

Changing Faces
1–2 Junction Mews
London W2 1PN
Tel: 020 7706 4232
www.changingfaces.co.uk

This is an excellent organisation that promotes the wellbeing of people affected by a visible disfigurement. They have a series of very helpful leaflets and information about how to deal with staring and teasing, as well as running workshops for young people and their families.

Teasing and bullying

Kidscape
2 Grosvenor Gardens
London SW1W 0DH

Tel: 020 7730 3300
www. kidscape.org.uk

This organisation was set up to help children who were being bullied and it campaigns for bullying to be taken seriously. It can provide some excellent clear material for children and young people, as well as their families, and also some excellent training packs for teachers.

General support for parents

Parentline
Tel: 080 8800 2222
www.parentlineplus.org.uk

Information regarding benefits and financial support

The Benefits Agency
Benefit Enquiry Line
Tel: 0800 882 200

Information regarding allergies

The Anaphylaxis Campaign
PO Box 275
Farnborough
Hampshire GU14 6SX
Tel: 01252 542029
www.anaphylaxis.org.uk

Allergy UK
Deepdene House
30 Belgrove Road
Welling
Kent DA16 3PY
Tel: 020 8303 8525
www.allergyuk.org

Companies supplying bedding, clothing or other equipment for children with eczema and allergies

Medivac Health Care Ltd
PO Box 33348

NW11 6YP
Tel: 0845 130 6969
www.medivac.co.uk

Allergy Best Buys (formerly The Sounder Sleep Company)
Tel: 08707 455002
www.AllergyBestBuys.com

This company stocks bedcovers, cotton sleepsuits and sleeping bags. They also stock hand tally counters for the habit reversal techniques that are described in Chapter 4.

Cotton Comfort
PO Box 71
Carnforth
Lancs LA5 9YA
Tel: 01524 730093
www.eczemaclothing.com

Schmidt Natural Clothing
21 Post Horn Close
Forest Row
Sussex RH18 5DE
Tel: 01342 822169

Halmax Healthcare
Tremaine Green
Pelynt
Nr Looe
Cornwall PL13 2LT
Tel: 01503 220006

Silk Story
3 National Terrace
Bermondsey Wall East
London SE16 4TZ
Tel: 0800 0150874
www.silkstory.com

Organisations providing information relating to complementary medicine

British Complementary Medical Association
PO Box 5122
Bournemouth
BH8 0WG
Tel: 0845 345 5977
www.bcma.co.uk

British Acupuncture Council
63 Jeddo Road
London W12 9HQ
Tel: 020 8735 0400
www.acupuncture.org.uk

British Medical Acupuncture Society
Administrator, 12 Marbury House
Higher Whitley
Warrington
Cheshire WA4 4QW
Tel: 01925 730727
www.medical-acupuncture.co.uk

British Homeopathic Association and Faculty of Homeopathy
15 Clerkenwell Close
London EC1R 0AA
Tel: 020 7566 7800
www.trusthomeopathy.org

Register of Chinese Herbal Medicine
Office 5, Ferndale Business Centre
1 Exeter Street
Norwich
NR2 4QB
Tel: 01603 623994
www.rchm.co.uk

Recommended further reading

Eczema and Your Child: A Parent's Guide
Tim Mitchell, David Paige and Karen Spowart
Class Publishing, 1998

Atopic Skin Disease: A Manual for Practitioners
Christopher Bridgett, Peter Noren and Richard Staughton
Wrightson Biomedical Publishing Ltd, 1996

Eczema in Childhood: The Facts
David Atherton
Oxford University Press, 1994

Systematic review of treatments for atopic eczema
C. Hoare, A. Li Wan Po and H. Williams
Health Technology Assessment, vol. 4, no. 37, 2000

Managing behaviour

The New Toddler Taming: A Parent's Guide to the First Four Years
Dr Christopher Green
Vermillion, 2001

The Incredible Years: A Trouble-shooting Guide for Parents of Children Aged 3–8
Carolyn Webster-Stratton
Umbrella Press, Toronto, 1992

Raising Happy Children: What Every Child Needs Their Parents to Know from 0–7 Years
Jan Parker and Jan Stimpson
Hodder and Stoughton, 1999

Toddler Troubles: Coping with Your Under-5s
Jo Douglas
John Wiley & Sons Ltd, 2002

Index

John Wiley & Sons
publish a wide range of groundbreaking **books, journals** and **online resources**
in many areas...

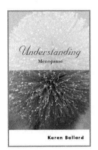
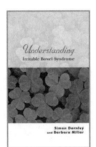
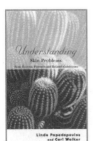
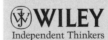